Disability
and Social Work Education:
Practice and Policy Issues

Disability and Social Work Education: Practice and Policy Issues has been co-published simultaneously as *Journal of Social Work in Disability & Rehabilitation,* Volume 6, Numbers 1/2 2007.

Disability
and Social Work Education:
Practice and Policy Issues

Francis K. O. Yuen, DSW
Carol B. Cohen, PhD
Kristine Tower, EdD
Editors

Disability and Social Work Education: Practice and Policy Issues has been co-published simultaneously as *Journal of Social Work in Disability & Rehabilitation,* Volume 6, Numbers 1/2 2007.

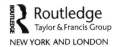

Routledge
Taylor & Francis Group
NEW YORK AND LONDON

First Published by

The Haworth Press, 10 Alice Street, Binghamton, NY 13904-1580 USA

Transferred to Digital Printing 2009 by Routledge
711 Third Ave, New York NY 10017
2 Park Square, Milton Park, Abingdon, Oxon, OX14 4RN

Routledge is an imprint of the Taylor & Francis Group, an informa business

First issued in paperback 2012

Disability and Social Work Education: Practice and Policy Issues has been co-published simultaneously as *Journal of Social Work in Disability & Rehabilitation,* Volume 6, Numbers 1/2 2007.

Library of Congress Catalog-in-Publication Data

Disability and social work education: practice and policy issues/ Francis K. O. Yuen, Carol B. Cohen, and Kristine Tower, editors.

    p. cm.

"Disability and social work education : practice and policy issues has been co-published simultaneously as Journal of social work in disability & rehabilitation, Volume 6, Numbers 1/2 2007."

Includes bibliographical references and index.
ISBN-13: 978-0-7890-2528-9 (hbk)
ISBN-13: 978-0-415-54269-2 (pbk)

   1. People with disabilities–United States. 2. Social work with people with disabilities–United States. I. Yuen, Francis K. O. II. Cohen, Carol B. III. Tower, Kristine.
HV1553.D545 2007
362.4'0453–dc22
                                                 2007015507

Disability
and Social Work Education:
Practice and Policy Issues

Francis K. O. Yuen, DSW
Carol B. Cohen, PhD
Kristine Tower, EdD
Editors

Disability and Social Work Education: Practice and Policy Issues has been co-published simultaneously as *Journal of Social Work in Disability & Rehabilitation,* Volume 6, Numbers 1/2 2007.

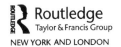

Routledge
Taylor & Francis Group
NEW YORK AND LONDON

First Published by

The Haworth Press, 10 Alice Street, Binghamton, NY 13904-1580 USA

Transferred to Digital Printing 2009 by Routledge
711 Third Ave, New York NY 10017
2 Park Square, Milton Park, Abingdon, Oxon, OX14 4RN

Routledge is an imprint of the Taylor & Francis Group, an informa business

First issued in paperback 2012

Disability and Social Work Education: Practice and Policy Issues has been co-published simultaneously as *Journal of Social Work in Disability & Rehabilitation,* Volume 6, Numbers 1/2 2007.

Library of Congress Catalog-in-Publication Data

Disability and social work education: practice and policy issues/ Francis K. O. Yuen, Carol B. Cohen, and Kristine Tower, editors.
    p. cm.
"Disability and social work education : practice and policy issues has been co-published simultaneously as Journal of social work in disability & rehabilitation, Volume 6, Numbers 1/2 2007."
Includes bibliographical references and index.
ISBN-13: 978-0-7890-2528-9 (hbk)
ISBN-13: 978-0-415-54269-2 (pbk)

    1. People with disabilities–United States. 2. Social work with people with disabilities–United States. I. Yuen, Francis K. O. II. Cohen, Carol B. III. Tower, Kristine.
HV1553.D545 2007
362.4'0453–dc22
                                                               2007015507

ABOUT THE EDITORS

Francis K. O. Yuen, DSW, ACSW, is Professor for the Division of Social Work at California State University, Sacramento. He is widely published in the areas of family health social work practice, disability, program evaluation, and services to refugees and immigrants. He is the editor for the *Journal of Social Work in Disability & Rehabilitation*. He has authored and edited many articles and books, including several for The Haworth Press, Inc., such as *International Perspectives on Disability Services: The Same but Different* (2004), and *Social Work Practice with Children and Families: A Family Health Approach* (2005).

Carol B. Cohen, PhD, LCSW-C, is Associate Professor for the MSW Program at Gallaudet University. Deafened as a young adult, she has spent several decades of her career advocating and providing services for deaf and hard of hearing populations. Dr. Cohen's publications and research interests are in disability, deafness, and clinical practice.

Kristine Tower, EdD, MSW, was Assistant Professor for the School of Social Work at the University of Nevada, Reno. Her research interests included persons with disabilities, sexuality, school social work, and consumer issues in social work. She was actively involved in disability-related concerns in the community and in local schools through legislative activity, training, advisory committees, assistive technology council, and public education. Dr. Tower passed away in October 2005.

Disability and Social Work Education: Practice and Policy Issues

CONTENTS

About the Contributors

Sandra J. Altshuler, PhD, LICSW, is Associate Professor in the School of Social Work at Eastern Washington University. Her research, teaching, and service all focus on supporting the health and well being of children, youth, and families, particularly so called "at-risk" youth (e.g., living in foster care, living with disabilities, living in a drug abusing environment). She has authored over 25 articles, book chapters, and technical reports that discuss the risk and protective factors that communities can address in supporting the needs of youth and families today.

Jeane W. Anastas, PhD, MSW, is Professor and Director of the PhD Social Work Program at New York University. She is the author of *Research Design for Social Work and the Human Services* as well as co-author of *Not Just a Passing Phase: Social Work with Gay, Lesbian and Bisexual People*. Dr. Anastas has authored numerous papers/articles in the areas of social work education, program evaluation, mental health and substance abuse and gay and lesbian issues. She is editor of the *Journal of Gay and Lesbian Social Services* and is on the editorial board of *Affilia: The Journal of Women in Social Work* as well as a consulting editor for *Social Work*.

Sharon Barnartt has a PhD from the Committee on Human Development at the University of Chicago and has taught in the Department of Sociology at Gallaudet University since 1980, except for one year when she had a Fulbright to teach at the University of Zimbabwe. Her research interests are in disability and deafness and the relationship of those to gender, socio-economic status, social movements, and social policy issues in the U.S. and developing countries. She is co-author of two books: *Deaf President Now: The 1988 Revolution at Gallaudet University* and *Disability Protests: Contentious Politics in the Disability Community*. She is co-founder and co-editor of the *Journal of Research in Social Science and Disability* and co-edited a special issue of *Disability Studies Quarterly* on deafness. Dr. Barnartt has published a number of articles and book chapters, and serves on the editorial board of the *Journal of Disability Policy Studies*. At Gallaudet University, she teaches many courses in sociology, including sociology of deafness, research methods and statistics, sociology of disability and medical sociology.

Carol B. Cohen, PhD, LCSW-C, is Associate Professor for the MSW Program at Gallaudet University. Deafened as a young adult, she has spent several decades of her career advocating and providing services for deaf and hard of hearing populations. Dr. Cohen's publications and research interests are in disability, deafness, and clinical practice.

Elizabeth Eckhardt, PhD, LCSW, is Project Director of Deaf Research at National Development and Research Institutes, Inc. Her previous related research includes the development of surveys in American Sign Language to study substance use, tobacco use, mental health, and HIV. Dr. Eckhardt graduated from New York University's School of Social Work and her dissertation analyzed in depth interviews with Deaf adults conducted in ASL to study HIV related health behaviors.

Reiko Hayashi, PhD, MSW, is Associate Professor in the College of Social Work at the University of Utah. Her research interests include disability, aging, health, and international social work. She is a member of the Society for Disability Studies and ADAPT. She works with local and international disability advocacy organizations to change disability-related policies in order to improve the lives of people with disabilities.

Jane Hurst, PhD, is Chair of the Department of Philosophy and Religion at Gallaudet University, the world's premier university for deaf, hard of hearing, and hearing impaired students. She has taught at Gallaudet University for over 25 years. Dr. Hurst received her PhD at Temple University, learning the skills of inter-cultural understanding and communication which has served her well as a hearing person whose professional life involved being a participant-observer in the Deaf world. Her research interests include new religious movements, religion and homophobia, and religion and disability.

Diane W. Keller, PhD, LSW, is Associate Professor in the School of Social Work at Marywood University. Her interests include program development and evaluation, and research related to children and adolescents with disabilities and their families. In addition, she is currently the administrator of the University Office for Research and Community Collaboration.

Nancy L. Mary, DSW, is currently Professor in the Department of Social Work at California State University at San Bernardino. She teaches policy and community practice, and has taught courses in introductory social work and social work with people with disabilities. Prior to pursuing an academic career, she received training in disabilities as an MSW student at UCLA Neuropsychiatric Institute's interdisciplinary Mental Retardation Program. Her primary practice experience has included program development, evaluation, and organizational development at Harbor Regional Center for People with Developmental Disabilities in the South Bay area.

Teresa Mason, PhD, MSW, is Associate Professor and Co-Director of the MSW program at Gallaudet University. She received her MSW from Gallaudet University in 1992 and her PhD from the University of Maryland in 2000. Dr. Mason's publications and research interests include measurement of ASL-translated scales, and mental health and public health services for deaf individuals.

Randall R. Myers, PhD, LCSW-C, is an international consultant on policy and mental health programs for Deaf and Hard of Hearing individuals. He is the editor of the Standards of Care for the Delivery of Mental Health Services to Deaf and Hard of Hearing Persons and continues to advocate to Deaf and Hard of Hearing individuals by serving as Chair of the Mental Health Committee of the National Association of the Deaf. Dr. Myers is a clinician as well as policy maker who has published numerous policy and procedure documents for several states focusing on accessibility issues.

Donna M. Napolitano, AA, is a published poet and employed part time at home for a beekeeper. She sustained a spinal cord injury at the c 5-6 level in 1975 resulting in quadriplegia. Her initial rehabilitation was at Rusk Institute in NYC in 1976. Ms. Napolitano received her AA degree at Central Florida Community College in 1998.

Cathy Orzolek-Kronner, PhD, LCSW, is Assistant Professor and Program Director in the Department of Social Work at McDaniel College. Her research interests include grief and loss, physical disabilities and mental health. Dr. Orzolek-Kronner has published journal articles in the areas of eating disorders and attachment, and EAP services to individuals who have multiple handicaps. Prior to her faculty position, Dr. Orzolek-Kronner spent over a decade practicing clinical social work.

Jean A. Pardeck, MEd, is a Reading Specialist in private practice. She is the co-author (with her husband John T. Pardeck) of several books including *Children in Foster Care and Adoption: A Guide to Bibliotherapy*, *Bibliotherapy: A Clinical Approach for Helping Children*, and *Bibliotherapy: A Guide for Using Books in Clinical Practice*. She has published extensively on the topic of bibliotherapy, in academic journals such as *School Counselor*, *Social Work in Education*, and *Early Child Development and Care*. She serves as the Associate Editor of the *Journal of Social Work in Disability & Rehabilitation*.

John T. Pardeck, PhD, LCSW, was Professor Emeritus in the School of Social Work at Missouri State University. He was an advocate for persons with disabilities and for interpreting the Americans with Disabilities Act to both private and public sector organizations. Dr. Pardeck was the author of *Social Work After the Americans With Disabilities Act: New Challenges and Opportunities for Social Service Professionals*. He also authored, co-authored, edited or co-edited 25 books, including *Family Health*, *Family Health Social Work Practice: A Macro Level Approach*, *Using Books in Clinical Social Work Practice*, *Children's Rights: Policy and Practice*, and *Social Work: Seeking Relevancy in the Twenty-First Century*. Dr. Pardeck published over 100 articles on disabilities and related topics in academic journals that included *Social Work*, *Child Welfare*, *Families in Society,* and *Research on Social Work Practice*. Until the time of his death, Dr. Pardeck was Editor-in-Chief of the *Journal of Social Work in Disability & Rehabilitation*.

Ashleigh Smith, MSW, recently graduated from the University of Houston Graduate College of Social Work with a Master of Social Work. She concentrated on politics, including policy analysis, empowerment, advocacy, and lobbying. She received her Bachelor of Arts in Social Work from Gallaudet University in 2004. Ashleigh participated in an effort to rally support for the ratification of the United Nations Convention on the Rights of Persons with Disabilities. She is passionate about the welfare of children, particularly those who are deaf and/or deaf-blind. She was inspired by a professor who was awarded the Nobel Peace Prize to pursue human rights activism as a potential part of her career. Ashleigh lives in Texas and is currently looking for employment in the political arena.

Diana Strock-Lynskey, MSW, is Professor of Social Work in the BSW Program at Siena College in Loudonville, NY. Her research and practice interests include gender equity, cultural diversity, disability, spirituality, death, loss, and grief, group work, organizational development, collaborative partnering, change management, public policy, advocacy, and activism. Her recent publications include, "The Case of Saundra Santiago," in R. Rivas and G. Hull (Eds.), *Case Studies in Generalist Social Work Practice and Entrepreneurship* and "The Mezzo/Macro Social Work Practitioner," in L. Grobman (Ed.), *More Days in the Life of Social Workers.*

Patricia Welch Saleeby, PhD, MSSA, is Assistant Professor in the School of Social Welfare at the University of Missouri-St. Louis. Her research interests include disability and health, social policy and social work practice, and international social work. She is a consultant for organizations such as the World Health Organization and American Psychological Association, and local disability organizations in the St. Louis area. Dr. Saleeby has contributed to the development of the International Classification of Functioning, Disability and Health and more recently the ICF Manual as the official NASW representative. She serves on the CSWE Commission on Disability and Persons with Disabilities and other disability-related boards and committees.

Preface:
Disability and Social Work Education

Carol B. Cohen, PhD, LCSW-C

> Vision is dynamic......
> It alters what its reflects:
> an individual's history, a particular time and place,
> an ideology, cultural identity
> the collective experience of a people
> It redefines and reshapes the larger world
> (Wells, 1993, p 83)

A vision can be more than a dream; a vision can be converted to public action, it can change the plight of an individual and it can change society as a whole. Social workers in the field of disability have a vision; this vision redefines the social construction of disability and incorporates the general principles of social justice for all.

This special volume was developed to enhance the knowledge, skill and value base of social work educators and students working with populations who interface with disability; addressing some of the gaps in the literature on social work education and disability. The contributors have extensive knowledge in the field of disability and have selected topics based on their extensive expertise in the field.

Carol B. Cohen, PhD, LCSW-C, Associate Professor, Department of Social Work Gallaudet University, 800 Florida Avenue NE, Washington, DC 20002 (E-mail: carol.cohen@gallaudet.edu).

[Haworth co-indexing entry note]: "Disability and Social Work Education." Cohen, Carol B. Co-published simultaneously in *Journal of Social Work in Disability & Rehabilitation* (The Haworth Press, Inc.) Vol. 6, No. 1/2, 2007, pp. xxix-xxxi; and: *Disability and Social Work Education: Practice and Policy Issues* (ed: Francis K.O. Yuen, Carol B. Cohen, and Kristine Tower) The Haworth Press, Inc., 2007, pp. xxi-xxiii. Single or multiple copies of this article are available for a fee from The Haworth Document Delivery Service [1-800-HAWORTH, 9:00 a.m. - 5:00 p.m. (EST). E-mail address: docdelivery@haworthpress.com].

Available online at http://jswdr.haworthpress.com
xxi

The basic tenets of social justice; accessibility to services and human rights as well as the social construction of disability that connotes inferiority are themes that are ubiquitous and addressed throughout most of the articles in this special issue. The authors integrate diverse perspectives for change on all levels (micro, mezzo and macro) of social work practice in order to address specific challenges in (work with disabled populations) the field of disabilities.

This special volume is a resource for social work educators, students as well as practitioners who want to embrace diverse and creative ways of integrating a generalist social work model in their work with various size systems that interface with disability. It is our aim to advance the training of social work students and practitioners who provide services for individuals, families, group and larger systems.

What are the challenges that social workers need to be aware of? Nancy L. Mary describes her educational experiences as a student who was exposed to the field of disabilities. Emphasizing the importance of education, she developed a model curriculum on disabilities that incorporates diverse perspectives of social work practice with individuals who have physical, cognitive and psychiatric disabilities. Sandra Altshuler emphasizes the importance of understanding and keeping abreast with policy changes in order to protect the legal rights of children for appropriate education. Knowledge of the historical changes and amendments to PL 94-142 are discussed in order for social workers to function as advocates for children and their families. This article focuses on the implication of Individuals with Disabilities Education Act (IDEA) policy and the ramifications for social workers in their attempts to advocate for adequate and appropriate education for children. Principles of policy and its implications for social action is further expanded by Reiko Hayashi who uses the bill known as MiCASSA (Medicaid Community Attendant Services and Supports Act) to highlight the importance of empowerment civil rights of disabled individuals to have access to community living. In her explanation of the grass roots history of the disability-rights movement that has led to the development of MiCASSA bill, she provides vivid examples of how disabled individuals have taken social action using Section 504 of the Rehabilitation Act, the Americans With Disabilities Act and the Supreme Court's Olmstead Decision to act as change agents in order to secure basic rights such as housing and medical care.

How do social work educators make accommodations necessary to teach social work students who are disabled? Ashleigh Smith, a deaf blind student, and Teresa V. Mason, her teacher, share their experiences in order for the reader to gain knowledge and insight into the academic process of helping students who are disabled achieve their academic goals.

Moving to the work setting, Jean A. and John T. Pardeck detail the historical and essential components of the Americans with Disabilities Act, noting key decisions made by the Supreme Court. Specific techniques/strategies for advocacy on the macro level are expatiated in order for social workers to facilitate accessibility and equal rights in the work environment. Randall R. Myers enhances one's knowledge of macro approaches by using his experience of development of the Standards of Care for the Delivery of Mental Health Services to Deaf and Hard of Hearing Persons to expound on various strategies of intervention for macro change.

Diana Strock-Linsky and Diane W. Keller provide a historical overview of family policy and practice as it relates to children and adolescents who are disabled. This article focuses on a family centered practice model of social work practice to address the diverse needs of children and adolescents.and highlights the diverse roles of social worker as advocate, collaborator, team member and family resource. As one approaches adulthood, the focus on intervention may change as exemplified in adult cases described by Donna Napolitano and Carol B. Cohen The biopsychosocial framework is used as an assessment tool to develop interventions focusing on adaptations/life choices that are necessary to adequately meet psycho/social/developmental needs and enhance the self esteem of individuals who are disabled. Cathy Orzolek-Kronner elaborates on the use of the therapeutic relationship, in particular the clinical issues that arise in her work as a disabled social worker, expanding on the use of psychodynamic and ecological approaches to social work practice. One's religious and spiritual beliefs can facilitate or hinder one's acceptance of oneself and one's disability. Jane Hurst outlines the therapeutic/value issues related to one's religious and spiritual belief and the interface with disability. Focus is placed on the expansion of one's knowledge of social workers to help clients develop adaptive religious and spiritual views.

Sharon N. Barnartt discusses disability protests and movements; both in respect to the objectives of the protest and as well as the implications those demands have on social work practice. Patricia Welch Saleeby shares her extensive work on the Capacity Approach and the International Classification of Functioning, Disability and Health which are used as tools to help social workers make accurate understanding of the client in an environmental situation. In hopes that our colleagues and students pursue research agenda in the field of disabilities, Elizabeth Eckhardt and Jeane Anastas provide basic guidelines for individuals who wish to undertake research about and with people who have disabilities.

REFERENCE

Wells, D. (1993). *We have a dream: African American visions of freedom.* New York: Carroll & Grat Publishers.

Acknowledgments

Francis Yuen is thankful for the teaching and support of his family. He wants to express his appreciation to the late Dr. John Terry Pardeck for his vision and support that made this special publication possible. He also would like to thank Dr. Roland Meinert who inspired the conceptualization of this project. Carol B. Cohen extends special gratitude to her family, especially her husband who has been an outstanding role model in adjusting to his disability. The editors appreciate the individual authors for their willingness to contribute to this special collection and share their academic and professional expertise with the readers. We are particularly thankful for the editorial assistance of Bernadine Bertrand for the initial copy and Jean Pardeck for her expert editing of the final manuscript. The editors are grateful for the support, patience, and expertise of the staff at The Haworth Press. Last but not least, we want to thank our students and clients. It is their insights, critiques, and encouragement that inspired us in the development of this special volume.

[Haworth co-indexing entry note]: "Acknowledgments." Co-published simultaneously in *Journal of Social Work in Disability & Rehabilitation* (The Haworth Press, Inc.) Vol. 6, No. 1/2, 2007, p. xxxiii; and: *Disability and Social Work Education: Practice and Policy Issues* (ed: Francis K.O. Yuen, Carol B. Cohen, and Kristine Tower) The Haworth Press, Inc., 2007, p. xxv. Single or multiple copies of this article are available for a fee from The Haworth Document Delivery Service [1-800-HAWORTH, 9:00 a.m. - 5:00 p.m. (EST). E-mail address: docdelivery@haworthpress.com].

Available online at http://jswdr.haworthpress.com
xxv

An Approach to Learning About Social Work with People with Disabilities

Nancy L. Mary

SUMMARY. The author shares some practice experience and personal reflection on her introduction to working with people with disabilities. Recognizing that the construct of "disability" is in the eye of the beholder, she shares an outline for one approach to an introductory course in working with people with physical, cognitive and developmental, and psychiatric disabilities. Common themes in practice and service delivery are discussed, as well as the unique role social workers can play in interagency collaboration. doi:10.1300/J198v06n01_01 *[Article copies available for a fee from The Haworth Document Delivery Service: 1-800-HAWORTH. E-mail address: <docdelivery@haworthpress.com> Website: <http://www. HaworthPress.com> © 2007 by The Haworth Press, Inc. All rights reserved.]*

KEYWORDS. Developmental disabilities, social work with disabilities, course on disabilities, clinical and social issues

---

Nancy L. Mary, DSW, is Professor, Department of Social Work, California State University-San Bernardino, 5500 University Parkway, San Bernardino, CA 92407, USA (E-mail: nmary@csusb.edu).

[Haworth co-indexing entry note]: "An Approach to Learning About Social Work with People with Disabilities." Mary, Nancy L. Co-published simultaneously in *Journal of Social Work in Disability & Rehabilitation* (The Haworth Press, Inc.) Vol. 6, No. 1/2, 2007, pp. 1-22; and: *Disability and Social Work Education: Practice and Policy Issues* (ed: Francis K. O. Yuen, Carol B. Cohen, and Kristine Tower) The Haworth Press, 2007, pp. 1-22. Single or multiple copies of this article are available for a fee from The Haworth Document Delivery Service [1-800-HAWORTH, 9:00 a.m. - 5:00 p.m. (EST). E-mail address: docdelivery@ haworthpress.com].

Available online at http://jswdr.haworthpress.com
doi:10.1300/J198v06n01_01

"WHAT AM I DOING HERE?"

Here I was at my first field placement in my MSW Program, doing an internship in community organization at a local regional center for people with developmental disabilities. This setting was one of 21 such centers in the state, set up as the primary coordinator of services for people with developmental disabilities. With next to no experience working with people with disabilities, I thought to myself, "What am I doing here?" It was my first day. But, to my surprise and delight, the receptionist had my name on the staff telephone list! They were actually expecting me! I had my own desk filled with supplies, a note of welcome attached to a bud vase with a lovely rose, and a weekly outline for my orientation on the desk. Well . . . someone is ready!!

In the two weeks that followed, I went to meetings, accompanied case managers on their visits, and visited programs. And I met people with what appeared to me to be horrendous disabilities in all kinds of living arrangements. I almost shuddered as I hurried by a toddler with an enormous head in a stark crib in what was then referred to as a "state hospital." I couldn't speak. I wondered, "What am I doing here?" I visited a small home with a young adult male with a "dual diagnosis" of autism and bi-polar disorder who, upon my arrival, moved quickly to a corner of the living room and started slapping his helmet with his hand, rocking to and fro. I asked myself, "What is he doing here?" I visited a young woman "artist" in a community-based program in a neighborhood much like my own, whose speech was slurred and who had to be wheeled around in her wheelchair and helped to eat and drink. This woman, I was told, had sold several of her batiks and the staff was hoping to open a gallery to showcase her work, alongside with other clients' art. I don't think this last bit of information computed for me; all I could do was stare at her. "How is this possible?"

As the weeks progressed, it became clearer why I was there. I observed the quality and focus of the interactions between the professional staff and the clients. "Shadowing" a social worker at a large residential facility for people with multiple needs including health care, I watched her intervene, amid all of the medical jargon focused on the young Hispanic woman's deficits. Not derailed, she skillfully persisted with questions such as "What things CAN she do by herself?" and "Is she being helped to learn to brush her teeth?" and "Is she being assisted in meeting other residents who speak Spanish at mealtime rather than eating alone?" Hmmmm. . . . Different focus. Language. Strengths. Self-determination.

I sat in on a somewhat disorganized school IEP meeting with many professionals hastily reporting on a child in a special education class. Time was limited. Professionals were clearly in charge. The case manager (a social worker) attempted several times to get some opinions from the family. Time and again they were interrupted. Finally she said, "I know you're in a time crunch here, but I don't think we've had a chance to really hear from Mr. And Mrs. Freeman." Though resisted by the principal, the social worker then helped the parents set up separate meetings with several professionals to go over individual tests and to give their opinions about their child. Hmmmm . . . she's good! Start where the clients are. Make sure their rights are upheld in the process through advocacy and empowerment.

Then I observed a "behavioral funding" meeting. Gregory was being referred for in-home behavioral intervention for his aggressive behaviors. The psychologist agreed that the request made by the case manager for an in-home behavioral program was a good one for the child. Then the social worker spoke up. "Down the line, this could be very useful. But right now this family has major pressing needs. Dad has disappeared. Grandma is Mom's support now. They have no income, and Greg's mom is involved in a child abuse investigation, as they think Dad is abusing the older daughter. This family is chaotic as the moment. They are not ready for behavioral intervention." She then suggested that some casework needed to be done to stabilize the whole environment, before involving the family in an intervention plan focusing on the child that they probably could not carry out. Hmmmm . . . she sees the bigger picture. The family and the environment.

For me, this placement became the learning lab for the values and principles of social work I was studying in class. It fit! The service philosophy and interactions between the providers and the clientele were congruent with what I was learning about social work. Everyone is unique and can grow. People need advocacy when systems and professionals are not accessible. Relationships are paramount. You don't "do to or for" people. You listen and work with them. I knew why I was in this community-based regional center working with people with disabilities.

That was 1975. Systems and times change. But some things stay the same. People with disabilities want to be treated normally, to "obtain an existence as close to the normal as possible" (Wolfensberger, 1972).

WHAT IF IT HAPPENED TO YOU?

At a recent trip to a midwestern state fair a 35-year-old man with Downs Syndrome was not allowed to ride on a roller coaster unless he had the companionship of an adult without disabilities. Children as young as 7 were riding the roller coaster alone while this gentleman, who could independently navigate the metropolitan bus system, was told he was too incompetent to ride without supervision. At the same fair, a friend of his with cognitive disabilities was not served beer at a stand because his form of identification was the State issued ID and not a driver's license.

Social workers have a professional calling: to work with people who are vulnerable. Our Code of Ethics, our history of advocacy, and our challenge to intervene across systems make us critical assets in the lives of people who need help realizing their own dreams. The purpose of this article is to briefly introduce the topic of disabilities and to share a course in social work with people with disabilities. An approach to service needs will follow. Common issues and social work roles will then be discussed, with particular attention to an evolving area of social work expertise: interagency collaboration.

WHO ARE THE "DISABLED?"

All of us may become disabled, especially if we live a long life. Some of us are born with or experience disability in childhood. Most of us in the United States, due to better medical care, the wonders of science, and increased longevity, will become more familiar with disability as we age. Life with serious illnesses such as AIDS and chronic impairments such as arthritis is increasingly feasible. The 1990 U.S. Census Bureau and the Center for Disease Control (2001) estimate that between 53 and 54 million people in the US are currently experiencing limitations from a chronic health problem. Globally, natural catastrophes, civil wars and poverty make disability a worldwide phenomenon with global consequences (Albrecht and Verbrugge, 2000).

How are social workers involved? Over 50% of the 27,000 NASW members surveyed in the 1992 Social Work Labor Force Study reported their primary practice to be in the field of mental health (32.7%), medical clinics (12.5%), substance abuse (4.6%), gerontology (2.7%), or other area of disability (.5%). As social workers, we may personally experience disability and we will undoubtedly become familiar with physically and socially disabling conditions in a significant number of individuals in the course of our social work career.

As the result of the disability rights movement in the 1960s and 1970s, definitions have evolved, moving from a primarily pathology based definition to the recognition of environmental forces in a more social model of disability. In 1980 the World Health Organization attempted some clarification of "disability" with the following terms:

- "Impairment" Any loss of abnormality of psychological, physiological, or anatomical structure or function
- "Disability" Any restriction or inability of an individual to perform an activity within the range considered the norm for human beings
- "Handicap" A disadvantage or barrier by the environment or society that limits or prevents fulfillment of a normal role

The usefulness of a definition, of course, depends on who is using is for what purpose. The term "developmental disability," now considered a clinical term, evolved out of the need to capture the functional limitations of people with chronic conditions manifested before age five (developmental) with corresponding needs that would continue indefinitely. In California, the evolution of the definition and the service system was much affected by a political context. Initially targeted to people with "mental retardation," it changed in 1969 when powerful parent groups representing family members with similar needs began pounding on the doors for entrance. In 1973 regional centers for people with "developmental disabilities" opened those doors to people with cerebral palsy, autism, epilepsy, and other neurologically handicapping conditions.

Indeed, people with disabling conditions need labels to access service systems. But the term "disability" or "handicap" is also an identity. From the categories developed for thinking about disability, people choose what they want to be called based on how they are viewed by their peers, by mainstream society and by other disability groups. For many years people with developmental disabilities have wanted to be known as "people first," e.g., a person with cerebral palsy, as it emphasizes that the disability is not inherent in or synonymous with the person. Each person is an individual first. However, an equally vocal group has more recently denounced this language as offensive, claiming that the term was coined by powerful non-disabled people, preferring the term disabled people, which emphasize minority group identity politics (Albrecht, Seelman, and Bury, 2001).

As social workers, we need to understand the terms and use the right ones with the right groups to help people with disabling conditions get what they need. This demands familiarity with legal definitions for benefit systems, institutional jargon for services, and the meaning and definition of each individual's own identity and culture. Culture is complex.

For example, the meaning, causality, and prognosis for someone with "mental retardation" to a North Indian Hindu immigrant may be quite different than the meaning to most people in the United States. As one Hindu elder participant in one study described, "Someone has disability in this life because of something from a past life," he said, "and someone will have disability in a future life because of something in this life. It is very simple" (Gabel, 2004).

Since the 1970s people with disabilities have become politicized, worldwide, celebrating a positive identity and consciousness of their own "disability culture" (Barnes and Mercer, 2001). In the United States, Fine and Asch (1988) found that 74% of Americans with disabilities report a sense of common identity. But this cultural identity has also divided people with disabling conditions. Some have expressed that, with greater societal awareness and acceptance of inclusion, a separate identity movement would be counterproductive. Others, such as a portion of the deaf community, feel that "deaf pride," similar to the experience of black people or gays and lesbians, translates a private sphere of life into a positive public affirmation (Barnes and Mercer, 2001). In the latter culture, this has included a resistance to cochlea implants, assimilation, and genetic screening to identify and terminate a fetus with a likely hearing impairment.

Thus, understanding the evolution of the construct of "disability culture" is important for social workers (Tower, 2003; Barnes and Mercer, 2001; Davis, 1995; Mackelprang and Salsgiver, 1999; Wang, 1993). Of course, we cannot know all there is to know about the variety of ethnicities, religions, and other cultural groups through reading alone. We find our about how people see themselves and their culture by listening, observing, and asking them about how they view themselves and their world.

A COURSE IN SOCIAL WORK
WITH PEOPLE WITH DISABILITIES

There are many ways for a social work student to learn about working with people with disabilities, but the best way, of course, is to do it. That is, have an internship or service learning experience, where you can interact with people and service systems, read about them, and then process and integrate the two. What follows is one attempt I have made in a more traditional elective course. This course would, indeed, be strengthened if taken concurrently with a field placement or with a service-learning component in the course itself.

Not strictly a direct practice class, it first provides a context for practice in examining the sociological construct of disability, then frames practice from a bio-psycho-social perspective of the social worker, and explores some consumer perspectives on their own disabling conditions. The course then moves to the macro arena, and explores service delivery models and the role of the social worker within the models. Working within a ten-week timeframe, practical decisions were made on the scope of disabling conditions. Although chronic health conditions such as arthritis, diabetes, heart disease, and AIDS, are important areas to explore, time constraints led to a focus on three primary areas of disability: physical disabilities, developmental and cognitive disabilities, and psychiatric disabilities. The following outlines the course content (for further resources see the Appendix):

Unit I: Overview and Definitions (Week 1)

A. Course framework
B. Definitions of disability (e.g., diagnostic, legal, social)
C. History and models (e.g., medical, developmental, support; educational, vocational, psychiatric, social service)

Unit II: Perspective on Disability (Weeks 2-3)

A. The sociology of disability, stigma, and culture
B. Bio-psycho-social-environmental model of social work
C. Perspectives of disabled people (their own voices)

Unit III: Working with People with Physical Disabilities (Weeks 4-5)

A. Definitions, specific populations, e.g., deaf and hard of hearing; persons with mobility disabilities; persons with visual disabilities and blindness.
B. Practice issues and use of case studies (social work roles)
C. Service models (e.g., medical vs. vocational), case management, and independent living movement

Unit IV: Working with People with Developmental and Cognitive Disabilities (Weeks 6-7)

        A. Definitions, specific populations (e.g., autism, epilepsy; learning disabilities, attention deficit disorder)
        B. Practice issues and use of case studies
        C. Service models (e.g., evolution of regional center system in CA; education for all handicapped children; application of case management

Unit V. Working with people with Psychiatric Disabilities (Weeks 8-9)

        A. Definitions: Use of DSM IV, chronic mentally ill, mental health of special population groups (e.g., homeless, ethnic minorities, children)
        B. Practice issues and use of case studies
        C. Service models e.g., evolution of deinstitutionalization, the "clubhouse" model, consumer movement

Week 10: Students share what they learned with other class members

Individualized assignments can help students learn more about a particular set of disabling conditions and service systems. However, there are some common issues and roles that social workers need to explore relevant to their work with any group of people encountering disability.

COMMON THEMES IN PRACTICE AND SERVICE DELIVERY

Clinical Issues

Unfortunately, a common pervasive issue in working with people with disabling conditions is that of stereotyping and discrimination. Fine and Asch (1988) identify five myths that people in general attribute to persons with disabilities. Briefly they are: (1) disability is the driving force in their lives, which victimizes and limits them (2) people, not the physical or social environment, are generally the cause of their own disability (3) people with disabilities can never be in control of their lives (4) disability is the center of their being which defines all of their reference groups and their roles and (5) help is always needed and always appreciated. These myths help perpetuate the resulting discrimination which occurs in relation to physical and social isolation, lack of physical access to their environment, and lack of access to service systems. Thus, the roles of educator and advocate are key for social workers.

We should also be aware that there are some differences in issues related to the onset of the disability. A middle-aged couple is told that their only child, a three-year-old, has autism. A nineteen-year-old man headed for college on a basketball scholarship has a motorcycle accident and no longer walks; he is learning to use a wheelchair for mobility. A fifty-six-year-old female college professor with diet-controlled diabetes is told that what she thought were cataracts are now being called diabetic retinopathy. Each of these people will have different clinical needs; some of these are related to the onset and expected life course of the disability. Rolland (1989) identifies the following four distinctions relevant to the adaptation of the individual and the family to a disability: onset, course, lifespan, and incapacitation. Onset, for example can be acute and traumatic as a result of an injury or it can be gradual such as Alzheimer's. The course of the disability can be predictably progressive, such as certain kinds of cancer, constant, such as blindness, or it can be relapsing or episodic such as some kinds of mental illness. The lifespan may be predictably shortened, affecting changes in one's life goals. Incapacitation may vary greatly with individuals with the same condition, the causes of which are individual and environmental, complex and interacting.

Therefore, the social worker needs to understand the onset and course of the disability. This will enable them to anticipate the successes and losses experienced by the individual and assist them in coping with new changes and a new identity. For example, understanding phases of grief (Parks, 1983) and the awareness of the concept of "chronic sorrow" (Olshansky, 1962) may help a family in the initial reactions to a diagnosis of a disability in a child. It may help explain the continuing disappointment parents may re-visit, at every major life stage, as they adjust their expectations from those of parents of a normally developing child.

Understanding life cycle development of people with disabilities is not easy if one turns to prominent theories of human development, which in large part neglect the healthy development of persons with disabilities. Maas' (1984) approach to life cycle development, concerned with the interaction between people and their environments, and Mackelprang and Salsgiver's (1999) life stage development approach within the context of disability are useful theories for understanding development of people with disabilities. For example, a normal adolescent develops a sense of personal identity and independence separate from her parents. If parents provide physical caregiving of the adolescent, feelings of ambivalence and conflict can occur when the teenager is reliant on the parents, but resents the need for them to care for her intimate needs (Mackelprang and Salsgiver, p. 69). Awareness of such conflicts can help social workers help families navigate life's course with a family member who is disabled.

Social workers must honor the pain and disappointment individuals and families encounter related to the losses, constraints, compromises, and battles experienced as a result of a disability. Social workers must also honor the dignity of risk of every striving growing individual. That is, they must help people with disabilities and their family members fight the over protectiveness that naturally occurs, which is not unique to families of individuals with disabilities. No one wants their child or sibling to experience pain, suffering, or possible death if they can prevent them from dangerous or harmful circumstances. If we follow this instinct to its logical end, however, the freeways would be barren (which, speaking as one who is a long distance commuter, might not be a bad thing!). There is something within every parent of a fifteen-year-old which says "the idea of my child barreling down the highway at 70 MPH in this 2000 pound piece of sheet metal is unfathomable." But lo and behold, when their offspring turns sixteen, most parents undergo one of the most difficult trials of self-determination and you-me differentiation imaginable. We let them take the wheel. We allow them the dignity of risk. It is this kind of struggle that social workers must help individuals and parents wrestle with, again and again, so that people with disabilities can take risks to become all that they desire. Listening to people with disabilities and their loved ones and then negotiating a quality of life that is rich, rewarding and sometimes dangerous, is a big part of social work.

People are social animals: friendships and interpersonal relationships are important in the lives of all people. However, studies have concluded that people with mental retardation are "the most socially invisible of all people with disabilities" (Smith and Anton, 1997, p. 398). Similarly, a high degree of social rejection of persons with mental illness was also found in a study that compared reactions to the behaviors of individuals with a label of mental illness and those labeled physically ill (Socall and Holtgraves, 1992). The implications of these findings are that if individuals are perceived as dangerous or disorderly, the willingness of non-disabled people to interact and pursue interpersonal relationships is compromised. Ravuad and Stiker (2001), in their discussion of the social processes of inclusion and exclusion point out the important interplay between the workplace and the fragility of relationships. When the two processes of unemployment and the loss of relationships occur simultaneously, the loss is one of "social bond." The problem of exclusion today may be as much a problem of broken social bonds as it is a problem of poverty. Substantial populations are at constant risk of finding themselves removed from what constitutes the very basis of social belonging, that is, "exchange" (Socall and Holtgraves, 1992, p. 496).

In this society meaningful activity is work or school. Students are learning to become future citizens and workers, and employees are contributing to the wealth of the society. But apart from these functions is the importance of the social space created by these institutions wherein friendships, role models and companionships are created. Perhaps the most important challenge of the social worker is to help individuals with disabilities connect with others to create social bonds and social supports, which enhance their quality of life.

Finally, the topic of sexuality must be addressed. The reason it must be discussed is, as a society, we have an unhealthy attitude toward it. The media flaunts it, yet we avert our eyes, especially in the world of disability. But we are neglectful of an important aspect of human development if, as social workers, we do not talk with individuals and families about sexuality as it relates to their particular disabling condition. In their article "Sexuality and Disability," Keller and Buchannan (1993) discuss some practical solutions to common problems, focusing primarily on individuals with physical disabilities. My own work has been with people with developmental disabilities and their parents and care providers. In talking about sexuality, friendships, intimacy, and personal safety, I have learned the following: Sexuality is often framed as a problem or "risky business." It is difficult and sometimes dangerous to separate the "nuts and bolts" from the social context. Because a discussion of sexuality has to begin with the individual and their significant others, I have come up with several principles in support of people's social and sexual development. I believe these are workable with all people, disabled and nondisabled:

- Listen and value what the person wants to be as a sexual human being
- Reinforce them as capable of meaningful intimacy–the sky's the limit
- Structure positive, not negative strategies for expressing sexuality in a relationship context
- Give people control over their own lives
- Model a positive view of yourself and others as sexual human beings

WHAT DO PEOPLE WITH DISABILITIES NEED?
A PERSPECTIVE ON SERVICE

What do all people need to live healthy happy lives? They need safe housing and food, an income, health care, meaningful activity (paid or unpaid work or school), and opportunities to interact with friends.

As agency based social workers, your particular organization has a mission, and the degree to which you are able to serve the whole person and the above needs depends greatly on the mission and model of the organization. If, for example, you work in a hospital, your service model is a medical one, and your responsibilities may be time limited, focusing on assisting the patient in establishing aftercare and an environment that will keep them as healthy as possible. If you work in a regional center for people with developmental disabilities, your service model is case management, and you may be able to assist and broker supports and services that cut across all of the above mentioned human needs, within a much longer timeframe. To further explore service models related to disability see Chapter One in Mackelprang and Salsgiver (1999).

The history of the treatment and service models for people with disabilities in the United States is well documented (Braddock and Parich, 2001; Mackelprang and Salsgiver, 1999; Berkowitz, 1987; Mary, 1998). In a nutshell, it begins in the colonies with the "moral model" wherein people with disabilities were seen as sinful and needing blessing or punishment. As we became more enlightened we moved to a "deficit model" and looked to genetics to explain disability. In the context of a eugenics movement, we advocated prevention of the conceptualization of people with disabilities an institutionalization for those who were already disabled. As science advanced in the 20th century, we embraced a "medical model" wherein we tried to cure the disease or contain those who could not be cured via custodial care. The Civil Rights movement led to the evolution of a "social/minority model" for many disenfranchised groups, as the social and policy environment was targeted as needing change. Today, though the times are not as ripe for social change as in the 1960s, we are experiencing what French and Swain (2001) describe as "the growth of a disabled people's movement and the establishment of a social model in the reconstruction of power relations and structures in professional-disabled people relations" (p. 734). This has resulted in such trends as service delivery by peers (Solomon, 2004); integrated education services (Haring, Haring and Lovett, 1992), person-centered planning (Mount, 1992, O'Brien and Lovett, 1992); growth of independent living centers (Braddock and Parish, 2001) and increasing popularity of vouchers or "direct payment" for disabled people (French and Swain, 2001).

What does this mean in terms of social work with people with disabilities? It means that the major "service" question has been reframed. The old question was, "What are the deficits and problems of this disabled person and what services are the 'best fit' for them?" The new question is, "What are your dreams and goals and what supports do you need to attain them?" This question, directed to the individual, is much more reflective of strengths and empowerment perspectives, valuing the unique person, and starting where the person is, all part of our Code of Ethics. When we are working with a 27-year-old male with a diagnosis of depression and mental retardation who is determined to be an airline pilot, our response is not "Wouldn't you like to try Goodwill Industries first?" Our response is to explore the "whys" of this dream. If we should discover that the real love is being around airplanes and airports, we can explore how that can happen. This could result in a job at the airport, a visit to or volunteer work at the aeronautical museum, or a match with a big brother who happens to be a pilot. The first question focuses on skill deficits and programs to develop or sustain them. The second on dreams and supports to reach them.

The other thing social workers must do, in considering the human needs of all people, the majority of whom are current or future taxpayers, is to start with the generics. That is, those services we all pay for, for all of us to use. If we continue the discussion from a "supports" frame of mind vs. one of "specialized, often segregated programs," we will find ourselves in the bigger generic picture. Litvak and Enders (2001) in their discussion of support systems note, "one of the problems with focusing primarily on an individual's disability is that professionals can forget that everyone, including people with disabilities, lives in a larger generic support envelope. Too often, the focus gets restricted to the part related to the 'special needs' relevant to disability" (p. 723). The generic big picture gets lost, e.g., public transportation, parks and recreation, senior centers. Restricting our thinking to specialized services often results in isolated support systems such as segregated housing and work training settings (sheltered workshops). Special Olympics would be more than happy to recruit, transport, and welcome Joey and his wheel chair, with open arms. But what he really wants to do is be a member of a local Boy Scout troop where he can go camping and earn merit badges. This means that, as social workers, we have to think outside the box, go where no one has gone before, and advocate for inclusion and against discrimination. Indeed, there are many challenging roles in social work with people experiencing disabilities.

PRACTICE ROLES

Unlike others, such as psychologists, social workers are unique human service professionals in our charge to intervene with systems at all levels. Thus, as generalist practitioners, we will find ourselves counseling, mediating, resource brokering, evaluating, advocating with individuals and families as well as across service systems on behalf of people with disabilities (Kirst-Ashman and Hull, 2002). Great job, eh? Never a dull moment! Beats a 50-minute hour (author's op ed). Particularly rewarding are roles that cut across small and large systems, such as the role of case manager. There are short term as well as comprehensive models of case management. Social workers will work within settings that have adopted one or another again depending upon their mission, their resources and their fit within the larger systems of service delivery to their clientele. Having said that, I would recommend a look at Rothman and Sager's *Case Management: Integrating Individual and Community Practice* (1998) for two reasons: (1) It is an extremely comprehensive discussion of the roles of a social worker and (2) It is focused on the needs of people who are "severely vulnerable" who will "require protracted and multifaceted services over a life time" (p. 3), such as elderly people, people with mental illness and developmental disabilities and people with physical disabilities.

I now want to spend some time discussing two roles I strongly believe are critical in working with people with disabilities: role modeling and interagency collaboration.

When I reflect on my own life, my successes have come, in large part, from my familial and social networks, my own perseverance, and from a host of environmental forces such as public and private resources that supported a working class female to pursue higher education. But the ones that have given meaning to my success and to my life are my role models. These mentors and cheerleaders knew I could get where I wanted to be and would not let me give up. Social workers with disabilities can be powerful forces in the lives of others with a condition and a society that throw hurdles in their path. Social workers with and without significant disabilities can play a vital role in connecting people, in person and electronically, to peer networks, support groups, self-help and self-advocacy groups, to those who have "been there." The history and successes of groups such as Disabled in Action, the National Alliance for the Mentally Ill, and People First are well documented; their stories are an inspiration to workers and clients alike. (Shapiro, 1993; Racino, 1999; Solomon, 2004; Dybwad and Bersani, 1996)

Collaboration: Buzzword of the New Millenium or Wave of the Future?

Social workers are taught to practice as members and facilitators of multi and interdisciplinary teams within their organization, for case conferencing and service coordination. Attention has also been paid in social work curriculum to working across organizational boundaries for resource development. What administrators and academics are now experiencing, however, is a need for social workers to play a role in what is loosely termed "interagency collaboration," to recruit new and unique organizational partners, structures and ventures (Mulroy, Nelson, and Gour, 2004). The reasons for this trend, occurring in business, government and private human services, are both local and global. They include the following: rapid economic and technological change, declining productivity and increased competition, blurring of boundaries between business, government and labor, decreasing federal investment in social programs, declining success in existing modes of problem solving (Gray, 1989, p. 29). A 1990 survey of state agencies serving children and families found that in 74% of the states, "coordination among agencies or departmental divisions is viewed as a major problem area, . . . policy makers throughout the country are calling for more collaborative responses to troubled children and families . . . and that the potential of collaboration is just beginning to be explored (Robison, 1990, pp. 20-21).

The literature in collaboration is new and rapidly evolving. Collaboration can be defined as "a process of joint decision making among key stakeholders of a problem domain about the future of that domain" (Gray, p. 227). It can occur among informal groups, businesses, public and private organizations at the local, state or national level. The result of these efforts, however, is always something new and, ideally, the process initiates a long-range commitment to problem solving within the domain. This may take the form of informal networks, committees, strategic alliances, joint ventures, or mergers (Backer, 2003). Studying collaboration has been a high priority of the Amherst H. Wilder Foundation. Mattessich, Murray-Close, and Monsey (2001), with the Wilder Research Center, reviewed the research literature on collaboration and, through an extensive meta analysis, identified twenty success factors from 40 case studies. These fell into six groups: (1) factors related to the environment and history of collaboration (2) membership characteristics (3) process and structure (4) communication (5) purpose and (6) resources. Backer, T. (2003) and associates have also looked at the evaluation process and tools for assessing collaborations, including a discussion of multicultural issues (Norman, 2003).

In a recent revision of the MSW Program at California State University, San Bernardino (Dept. of Social Work, CSUSB, 2003), the advanced core curriculum contains a course in interagency collaboration, focusing on process, skills, and the types of collaborations social workers may help develop in any field of practice. Though there are various models of collaboration, the process is clearly delineated in four stages in The *Collaboration Handbook* (Winer and Ray, 2001), which provides theory and a workbook most appropriate for MSW level students. Types of collaboration explored in this curriculum include the following: political advocacy (Gilson, 2004); social change (Roberts-DeGennaro and Mizrahi, 2004); community university partnerships (Cook, Bond, Jones, and Greif, 2002) and service learning (Mary and Davis, 2004); service integration (Kimmich, 1994; Mulroy, Nelson, and Gour, 2004); and corporate alliances (Austin, J., 2000).

Social workers who work with individuals with disabilities and their families have many inspiring collaboration examples to draw from to stimulate new programs and initiatives in any kind of organization. The following are just a few. Mount Hope, just one Community Development Corporation (CDC) in the South Bronx, partnered with the Mid Bronx Desperadoes Community Housing Corporation to develop an innovative child and family development program to help parents boost the development of at risk children by becoming more effective teachers of their toddlers. This partnership is modeled on a program brought to the United States from Israel in the 1980s (Schorr, 1992, p. 333). In Orlando, Florida, a disability rights activist contacted Valencia Community College and, in partnership with the college, the United States Department of Education, and IBM, with its contacts at Disney World, AT&T, Westinghouse, Sunbank and Red Lobster, established a business advisory council to examine employment in high tech fields. One result was the Center for High-Tech Training for Individuals with Disabilities, a non-profit program to prepare people with severe physical disabilities for challenging high tech careers (Hurley, 2002).

Health care, or the lack of it, is a major issue for people with disabilities in the United States. In St. Paul, Minnesota, two rehabilitation industries, Courage Center and the Sister Kenny Rehabilitation Institute created a voluntary managed health care system for people with disabilities. The pilot for AXIS Healthcare was developed with the help of the Center for Health Care Strategies and the Robert Wood Johnson Foundation, "to bring disability knowledge to the managed care industry" (NewsRx.com, 2004, p. 191). With 300 people enrolled as of the spring of 2004, the program has served people with spinal cord injury, traumatic brain injury, cerebral palsy and multiple sclerosis.

Education has moved beyond defining inclusion as classroom integration to one that involves the development of collaborations in the provision of integrated life long services. For example, at Butte College in California, adults with developmental disabilities take classes in functional reading, reading, arithmetic and other useful skills (HEATH, 1988). The ACCESS project in Ohio is a partnership between the University of Akron and Kennedy Foundation, to provide volunteers to teach community skills to elders with disabilities over the age of 60 (Stroud and Sutton, 1988).

Collaboration does not have to involve numerous partners. In Baltimore, The League at Camp Greentop, a branch of the League for People with Disabilities, contacted Andy Herbick with the Downtown Sailing Center to put together a "Sailing Saturday Spectacular" for children and families of individuals with a variety of disabilities. The event "immensely heightened leisure awareness" and "majority of the participants said they now felt more confident in pursuing new activities" (National Therapeutic Recreation Society, 2003, p. 103). Collaboration (and self determination!) always begins with one step. The literature is rich with examples of short term, more philanthropic events that evolve into "transactional" and sometimes into "integrative" relationships (see the story of Timberland in Austin, 2000, Chapter 1).

So, what is the role of social work in these collaborations? Does this mean we have to be experts in health care financing, housing, business, child development, or computers? No, of course not. We all have our own areas of expertise. Our role is to get those with a stake, an interest, curiosity, expertise, a need, to the table, talking to each other. That's what we are good at, right?! We know how to mediate the process in our work with family members, self help group members, organizational staff, and community members who have some reason to meet. We know how to help them find common ground, a vision for something better, and a reason to come back to work on it together. That's why social workers should be at the forefront of building interagency, intersector collaborations.

CONCLUSION

It is my hope that, through sharing some information and personal reflection, the reader has gained further insight into working with people with disabilities and a desire to explore this work further. If you are embarking on a path with the dream of being a social worker, I hope you will consider this: Let yourself be open to learning your profession's unique values, skills, and "people processes." These will enable you to have the privilege to work alongside people in need, individuals who also have dreams but are experiencing difficulties navigating their own paths due to their own disabilities and disabling environments. Finally, whether a student, practitioner, or educator, if you are not presently disabled, you may well be only temporarily able. The battles you choose to engage in on behalf of people with disabilities will ultimately result in a better life for all of us.

REFERENCES

Albrecht, G., Seelman, K., & Bury, M. (2001). The formation of disability studies. In G. Albrecht, K Seelman, & M. Bury (Eds.), *Handbook of disability studies* (pp. 1- 8). Thousand Oaks, CA: Sage.

Albrecht, G., & Verbrugge, I. (2000). The global emergence of disability. In G. Albrecht, R. Fitzpatrick, & S. Scrimshaw (Eds.) *The handbook of social studies in health and medicine* (pp. 293-307). Thousand Oaks, CA: Sage.

Austin, J. (2000). *The collaboration challenge.* San Francisco: Jossey Bass.

Backer, T. (Ed.) (2003). *Evaluating community collaborations.* New York: Springer Publishing Co.

Barnes, C., & Mercer, G. (2001). Disability culture assimilation or inclusion. In G. Albrecht, K Seelman, & M. Bury (Eds.), *Handbook of disability studies* (pp. 513-534). Thousand Oaks, CA: Sage.

Berkowitz, E. (1987). *Disability policy: America's programs for the handicapped: A Twentieth Century report.* Cambridge: Cambridge University Press.

Braddock, D., & Parish, S. (2001). An institutional history of disability. In G. Albrecht, K. Seelman, & M. Bury (Eds.), *Handbook of disability studies* (pp. 11-68). Thousand Oaks, CA: Sage.

Cook, D., Bond, A., Jones, P., & Greif, G. (2002). The social work outreach service within a school of social work: A new model for collaboration with the community, *Journal of Community Practice,* 10(1), 17-31.

Davis, L. J. (1995). *Enforcing normalcy: Disability, deafness, and the body.* London: Verso.

Dybwad, G., & Bersani, J. (1996). *New voices: Self-advocacy by people with disabilities.* Cambridge, MA: Brookline.

Fine, M., & Asch, A. (1988). *Women with disabilities: Essays in psychology, culture and politics.* Philadelphia, PA: Temple University Press.

French, S., & Swain, J. (2001). The relationship between disabled people and health and welfare professionals. In G. Albrecht, K. Seelman, & M. Bury (Eds.), *Handbook of disability studies* (pp. 734-753).Thousand Oaks, CA: Sage.

Gabel, S. (2004). South Asian Indian cultural orientations toward mental retardation, *Mental Retardation*, 42(1), 12-25.

Gilson, S. (2004). The underground advocates: Legislative advocacy for and with service users with disabilities. In D, Fauri, S. Wernet, & E. Netting (Eds.), *Cases in macro social work practice* (pp. 47-62). New York: Person Education.

Gray, B. (1991). *Collaborating: Finding common ground for multiparty problems.* San Francisco: Jossey Bass.

Haring, K., Haring, N., & Lovett, D. (1992). *Integrated lifecycle services for persons with disabilities.* New York: Springer-Verlag.

HEATH (1988). New alternatives after high school for persons with severe handicaps. *Information from HEATH, 7*(3), 3.

Hewitt, A., & O'Nell, S. (1998). Speaking up–Speaking out. Washington D.C.: The President's Committee on Mental Retardation.

Hurley, K. (2002). High-tech partnering leads to learning-centered curricula for individuals with disabilities, *New directions for community colleges*, No. 119.

Keller, S., & Buchanan, D. (1993). Sexuality and disability: An overview. In M. Nagler (Ed.), *Perspectives on disability* (pp. 227-234). Palo Alto, CA: Health Markets Research.

Kimmich, M. (1994). Collaboration in action. In V. Bradley, J. Ashbaugh, & B. Blaney (Eds.), *Creating individual supports for people with developmental disabilities*, (pp. 403-420). Baltimore: Paul Brookes Publishing Co.

Kirst-Ashman, K., & Hull, G. (2002). *Understanding generalist practice.* Pacific Grove, CA: Brookes/Cole.

Litvak, S., & Enders, A. (2001). Support systems: The interface between individuals and environments. In G. Albrecht, K. Seelman, & M. Bury (Eds.), *Handbook of disability studies* (pp. 711-733). Thousand Oaks, CA: Sage.

Maas, H. (1984). *People in contexts: Social development from birth to old age.* Englewood Cliffs, NJ: Prentice Hall.

Mackelprang, R., & Salsgiver, R. (1999). *Disability: A diversity model approach in human service practice.* Pacific Grove, CA: Brooks/Cole.

Mary, N. (1998). Social work and the support model of services for people with developmental disabilities, *Journal of Social Work Education, 34*(2), 247-260.

Mary, N., & Davis, T. (2004). Service learning and social work, manuscript in progress.

Mattessich, P., Murray-Close, M., & Monsey, B. (2001). *Collaboration: What makes it work.* St. Paul, MN: Amherst H. Wilder Foundation.

Mount, B. (1992). *Person-centered planning.* New York: Graphic Futures Inc.

Mulroy, E., Nelson, K., & Gour, D. (2004). Community building and family-centered service collaboratives. In M. Weil (Ed.), *The handbook of community practice* (pp. 460-476). Thousand Oaks, CA: Sage.

National Therapeutic Recreation Society (2003). SAIL: Soaring abilities in leisure, *Parks and Recreation*, September, 2003.

NewRx.com (2004). New program developed to bring disability knowledge to managed care industry, *Health and Medicine Week*, April 12, 2004.

Norman, A. (2003). Multicultural issues in collaboration: Some implications for multirater evaluation. In T. Backer (Ed.) *Evaluating community collaborations* (pp. 19-36). New York, NY: Springer Publishing Co.

O'Brien J., & Lovett, H. (1992). *Finding a way toward everyday lives: The contribution of person centered planning*. Harrisburg, PA: Pennsylvania Office of Mental Retardation.

Olshansky, S. (1962). Chronic sorrow: A response to having a mentally defective child. *Social Casework, 43*, 190-193.

Parks, R. (1983). Parental reactions to the birth of a handicapped child. In L. Wikler & M. Keenan (Eds.). *Developmental disabilities no longer a private tragedy* (pp. 96-101). Silver Spring, MD: NASW.

Racino, J. (1999). Self-advocacy, the independent living movement, and personal assistant services, In A. Racino (Ed.) *Policy, program evaluation and research in disability: Community support for all* (pp. 171-187). Binghamton, NY: The Haworth Press, Inc.

Raiff, N. (1993). *Advanced case management: New strategies for the nineties*. (Chapter 2, "The Advanced Case Manager: A Quality Approach to Best Practice," and Chapter 3 "Quality Standards of Case Management Practice: Cultural Competency, Consumer Empowerment, Clinical Case Management and Multidisciplinary Practice." Newbury Park: Sage.

Ravuad, J., & Stiker, H. (2001). Inclusion/exclusion: An analysis of historical and cultural meanings, In G. Albrecht, K. Seelman, & M. Bury (Eds.), *Handbook of disability studies* (pp. 490-512). Thousand Oaks, CA: Sage.

Roberts-DeGennaro, M., & Mizrahi, T. (2004). Coalitions as social change agents, In M. Weil (Ed.), *The handbook of community practice* (pp. 305-318).Thousand Oaks, CA: Sage.

Robison, S. (1990). *Putting the pieces together: Survey of state systems for children in crisis*. Denver: National Conference of State Legislatures.

Rolland, J. (1989). Chronic illness and the family life cycle, In B. Carter & M. McGoldrick (Eds.), *The changing family life cycle*. Boston: Allyn and Bacon.

Rothman, J., & Sager, J. (1998). *Case management: Integrating individual and community practice*. Boston: Allyn and Bacon.

Sands, R., & Angell, B. (2002). Social workers as collaborators on interagency and interdisciplinary teams, In K. Bentley (Ed.), *Social work practice in mental health: Contemporary practice in mental health*. Boston: Brooks/Cole.

Schorr, L. (1997). *Common purpose: Strengthening families and neighborhoods to rebuild America*. New York: Anchor Books.

Shapiro, J. (1993). *No pity: People with disabilities forging a new civil rights movement*. New York: Tomes Books.

Smith, J., & Anton, M. (1997). Laura Bridgman, mental retardation, and the question of differential advocacy. *Mental Retardation, 35*(5), 398-401.

Socall, D., & Holtgraves, T. (1992). Attitudes toward the mentally ill: The effects of label and beliefs. *The Sociology Quarterly, 33*, 435-445.

Solomon, P. (2004). Peer support/peer provide services underlying processes, results, benefits, and critical ingredients, *Psychiatric Rehabilitation Journal, 27*(4), 392-401.

Stroud, M., & Sutton, E. (1988). *Expanding options for older adults with developmental disabilities: A practical guide to achieving community access.* Baltimore, MD: Paul H. Brookes.

Tower, C. (2003). Disability through the lens of culture, in F. Yuen (Ed.). *International perspectives on disability services: The same but different* (pp. 5-22). Binghamton, NY: The Haworth Press, Inc.

U.S. Bureau of the Census. (1991). SIPP User's Guide 2nd ed. Washington D.C.: Author.

VanderSchie-Bezyak, J. (Jan-Mar 2003). Service problems and solutions for individuals with mental retardation and mental illness, *Journal of Rehabilitation, 69*(1), 53-59.

Walter, U. (2000, September). A template for family-centered interagency collaboration. *Families in Society: The Journal of Contemporary Human Services. 81*, 494-499.

Wang, C. (1993). Culture, meaning, and disability: Injury prevention campaigns and the production of stigma. In M. Nagler (Ed.) *Perspectives on Disability* (pp. 77-90). Palo Alto, CA: Health Markets Research.

Winer, M., & Ray, K. ((2000). *Collaboration handbook.* St. Paul, MN: Amherst H. Wilder Foundation.

Wolfensberger, W. (1972). *Normalization: The principle of normalization in human services.* Toronto, Canada: National Institute on Mental Retardation.

World Health Organization (WHO) (1980). International Classification of Impairments, Disabilities, and Handicaps: A Manual of Classification Relating to the Consequences of Disease. Geneva: Author.

doi:10.1300/J198v06n01_01

APPENDIX

COURSE FRAMEWORK

Types of Disabilities		
Physical	**Developmental and Cognitive**	**Psychiatric**
PERSPECTIVES How does the consumer and society define and perceive the disability?		
NEEDS/PRACTICE ISSUES What are the unique needs and practice issues for individuals and their families/ significant others?		
SERVICES What is (are) the service systems and models of service for individuals and families over the life span?		
DIRECT AND MACRO SOCIAL WORK ROLES What are the client/family directed and organizational/policy roles of social work within the various service models? What is the role of the consumer?		

Note on resources: This course outline is a condensed version of one of many complete course syllabi found in *Integrating Disability Content in Social Work Education: A Curriculum Resource* (2002). Alexandria Virginia: Council on Social Work Education. I would strongly recommend it, as it also contains readings, websites, and an annotated listing of popular films depicting characters with disability.

A note on texts: Two I have found most useful are the Makelprang and Salsgiver text and the Rothman text listed above in the bibliography.

Everything You Never Wanted to Know About Special Education . . . and Were Afraid to Ask (I.D.E.A.)

Sandra Altshuler

SUMMARY. Social workers who work with families and children are often unaware of the legal protections afforded to educational experiences for children, particularly to children with disabilities. Yet, all social workers, regardless of their practice setting, should be aware of the important educational rights to which children with disabilities and their families are entitled, as codified in the original legislation, P.L. 94-142, and its subsequent revisions. This legislation is currently entitled the "Individuals with Disabilities Education Act," or the "I.D.E.A." Provisions included in the I.D.E.A. are covered with which all states that receive federal educational funding are mandated to comply. Reviewed are the 13 "disabling conditions" that allow for students to qualify to receive special educational services, as long as one of the conditions is adversely impacting their educational success. It concludes with recommendations for social work advocacy regarding this legislation. doi:10.1300/J198v06n01_02 *[Article copies available for a fee from The Haworth Document Delivery Service: 1-800-HAWORTH. E-mail address:*

Sandra Altshuler, PhD, LICSW, is Associate Professor, School of Social Work, Eastern Washington University, 203 Senior Hall, Cheney, WA 99004 (E-mail: saltshuler@mail.ewu.edu).

[Haworth co-indexing entry note]: "Everything You Never Wanted to Know Special Education . . . and Were Afraid to Ask (IDEA)." Altshuler, Sandra. Co-published simultaneously in *Journal of Social Work in Disability & Rehabilitation* (The Haworth Press, Inc.) Vol. 6, No. 1/2, 2007, pp. 23-33; and: *Disability and Social Work Education: Practice and Policy Issues* (ed: Francis K. O. Yuen, Carol B. Cohen, and Kristine Tower) The Haworth Press, Inc., 2007, pp. 23-33. Single or multiple copies of this article are available for a fee from The Haworth Document Delivery Service [1-800-HAWORTH, 9:00 a.m. - 5:00 p.m. (EST). E-mail address: docdelivery@haworthpress.com].

KEYWORDS. Students with disabilities, the I.D.E.A., social work advocacy, educational rights

INTRODUCTION

The educational experiences of all children have significant impact on their overall well-being. Social workers who work with families and children are often unaware of the legal protections afforded to children, particularly to children with disabilities. All social workers who work with children and families, regardless of their practice setting, should be aware of the important educational rights to which children with disabilities and their families are entitled (Altshuler & Kopels, 2003).

The U.S. Congress enacted a veritable revolution in 1975, when it passed the Education for All Handicapped [note: I will use the term handicapped when it is historically accurate to do so] Act (P.L. 94-142), that provided sweeping rights to such students. Previous to the 1975 Act, schools were permitted to exclude students with any type of perceived handicaps, based on the principle of *in loco parentis*; e.g., that schools were free to make educational decisions acting in place of parents (Allen-Meares et al., 2000, and Washington & Welsh, 2000). Indeed, all that was required for exclusion was a request by a teacher, parent or administrator, stating that the child's handicap was making it too difficult either for the child or peers to learn, or for the teacher to teach. Further, there were no agreed-upon definitions about what a handicap was or was not; therefore, any person could claim that a student had a handicap, thereby justifying exclusion. These practices led to widespread private placements of students with handicaps if their parents could afford such services and widespread exclusion from accessing any benefits that public educational settings offer to all other students.

In 1975, P.L. 94-142 mandated that all handicapped children were entitled to receive special education and related services specifically designed to meet their needs and provided financial support to ensure its mandates. One of the primary purposes of the original legislation was to ensure that children with disabilities between the ages of 3 and

21 were not excluded from public schools. At the time of its passage, more than half of children with disabilities in the United States did not receive appropriate educational services, and one million children with disabilities were excluded entirely from the public school system [20 U.S.C. § 1400(c)(2)]. P.L. 94-142 also provided protections for the rights of parents, children, and educational institutions regarding its requirements. While P.L. 94-142 was designated as permanent legislation, Congress was required to reauthorize the federal financial support for it on a periodic basis (theoretically, every three years). During each reauthorization process, Congress was able to modify the requirements of the law.

Thus, P.L. 94-142 was reauthorized in 1990 and renamed the Individuals with Disabilities Education Act (P.L. 101-476), commonly referred to as the I.D.E.A. One of the major changes instituted in 1990 was the law's emphasis on comprehensive, coordinated, interagency early intervention services for infants and toddlers (Allen-Meares et al., 2000). The most recent amendments to the I.D.E.A. were adopted in 1999, and expanded definitions of disabilities, including addressing the needs of homeless children and children with disciplinary problems (Altshuler & Kopels, 2003). All of these changes, while significantly impacting the rights and protections of children with disabilities and their families, also retain the basic rights and protections that have been extended to them since the law's 1975 origin (Altshuler & Kopels, 2003). "P.L. 94-142" and the I.D.E.A. are terms often used interchangeably by professionals and lawmakers.

Throughout its history, states have developed policies to comply with the I.D.E.A. based on their varying interpretations of the law. Unfortunately, states' policies may not always comply with the requirements of the law. In fact, a recent study by the National Council on Disability found that all states are out of compliance with the law's requirements in some manner (National Council on Disability, 2000). Therefore, this article must, by necessity, cover the mandates found only in the *federal* law, and may not reflect individual states' interpretation and policy development. Because of the detail that can be included in every provision of this law, this article will review only the basic protections provided, including the legal definitions of educational handicaps, so that all social workers will be in a strong position of advocacy for their clients, no matter what setting they are placed. For more details about any of these provisions, the student is encouraged to review the law itself and its accompanying revisions.

Provisions of P.L. 94-142

Zero Reject/Child Find: One of the most important messages of P.L. 94-142 is that *all* children with disabilities fall within the provisions of the law. No child may be rejected or excluded from accessing education based upon the existence of a disability. Furthermore, P.L. 94-142 requires every state to identify, locate, and evaluate all children with disabilities residing in that state [34 C.F.R. § 300.125]. This "child find" principle applies to all children with disabilities, regardless of the severity of the disability or their attendance at private schools. In 1999, Congress clarified that the child find requirements also apply to highly mobile children with disabilities and specifically define highly mobile children with disabilities to include those who are migrant or homeless (Altshuler & Kopels, 2003). Congress also explicitly required that school districts take a more active role in searching out and finding these families and children, rather than leaving the burden of self-identification up to the families themselves.

Free and Appropriate Public Education (FAPE): The original law stated that children with disabilities are entitled to receive a free and appropriate public education, commonly referred to as a FAPE. As Altshuler and Kopels (2003) explain, the term FAPE means that special education and related services are provided at public expense and without charge to parents; meets State defined standards; includes education from preschool through high school; and are provided in conformity with an individualized education program [34 C.F.R. § 300.13].

Least Restrictive Environment (LRE): This provision of the law requires that students with disabilities receive a FAPE, to the maximum extent possible, with non-disabled, general education students (Allen-Meares et al., 2000). Special education services can be considered a continuum of services, from consultative services on one end, spanning to institutional care on the other end. The extent to which a student's day is restricted from the typical interactions with their non-disabled peers is how the level of environmental restriction is determined. The overall purpose of the LRE provision is to ensure that schools minimize the amount of time a student is not with their non-disabled peers.

Nondiscriminatory Evaluation (NDE): Children with disabilities were protected from nondiscriminatory evaluation through a requirement that a multidisciplinary team must complete a wide range of non-biased assessments specific to children's suspected disabilities before placement into special education can occur (Altshuler & Kopels, 2003). The NDE must be completed by professionals qualified and knowledgeable in the relevant disability being evaluated. The NDE cannot use a single assessment, or a single discipline, as a sole determinant for placement into special education; it must be comprised of a variety of valid, standardized, non-biased assessment instruments administered by more than one professional [20 U.S.C. § 1414 (b)]. Some states refer to the NDE as a case study evaluation ("CSE"). Regardless of its terminology, the NDE/CSE must be fully re-done every three years, to ensure continuing appropriateness of placement.

Multidisciplinary Team (MDT): The MDT, as defined, is comprised of a variety of professionals from a variety of disciplines, who administer and evaluate the standardized assessments for determining eligibility for special education placement. However, the MDT does more than simply assess and evaluate. The MDT attends meetings, often called Multidisciplinary Conferences (MDCs), at which eligibility, placement and educational decisions are made. As such, in addition to the professionals who are performing the evaluations, the MDT is comprised of at least one of the student's general education and special education teachers; a representative from the local educational administration (LEA) who is familiar with both the general curriculum and the available resources; and the student's parents [20 U.S.C. § 1414 (d)(1)(B)]. This is true regardless of the student's age (e.g., 3-21), although after age 14, it is expected that the student would also become a member of the MDT.

Individualized Education Program (IEP): A FAPE is ensured, and children with disabilities are protected from inappropriate educational services, by the mandate that schools must create an Individualized Educational Program. This plan, known as an IEP, is designed specifically for each student receiving special services, a plan that must be reviewed and rewritten yearly to reflect current functioning and progress toward educational goals (Altshuler & Kopels, 2003). As Turnbull and Turnbull (1998) delineate, the IEP is required to have a number of components [20 U.S.C. § 1414 (d)(1)(A)]:

1. A statement of students' present levels of educational functioning and how the disability impacts their ability to progress within the general curriculum;
2. A statement of measurable annual goals and short-term objectives that address the students' educational needs that result from their identified disability;
3. An outline of the specific special education services, related services, supplemental services, and program modifications that will

be made in order to achieve the measurable annual goals, including their frequency, duration and location;

4. Any modifications in standardized testing (while this is beyond the breadth of this chapter, it is important to point out that this provision in P.L. 94-142 is contradicted by provisions in the No Child Left Behind Act (P.L. 107-110), which specifically disallows any such exclusion or modification for students with disabilities) and how students will be appropriately assessed for educational progress;

5. A statement of how students' progress toward the annual goals will be measured and how their parents will be regularly informed; and

6. When students reach the age of 14 (and older), a statement of transitional service needs and agency linkages, if appropriate.

The 1990 Amendments that provided for early intervention services also revised requirements for an individualized educational program specifically designed for infants and toddlers. One revision was the requirement of an Individualized Family Service Plan (IFSP) that must be developed for any child identified with a disability younger than 5 years old. As the name indicates, the primary distinction between an IEP and an IFSP is the requirement that the family be included in any individualized program for such children [20 U.S.C. § 1436]. In addition, all IFSP's must define the specific steps involved in transitioning the child to their next educational setting.

Parent Involvement/Procedural Due Process: Every iteration of the I.D.E.A. from its inception has attempted to ensure parental involvement and participation in the special education process. Under the current law, a parent may be defined as a birth or adoptive parent, a legal guardian, a surrogate parent, or someone acting in the place of a parent (e.g., foster parents) [34 C.F.R. § 300.20]. The general idea (not the legal technicalities) of procedural due process has to do with fairness and the ability of the parents to legally disagree with decisions being made about their children. In effect, the federal government has defined exactly how state and local educational agencies must include parents throughout the entire process, and, the legal procedures by which parents can ensure that their, and their children's, rights are being protected. The I.D.E.A. delineates a series of requirements for State Educational Agencies (SEAs) to involve parents in decision-making about policies and procedures for special education. For example, all SEAs are required to create Advisory Panels for special education that are primarily comprised of parents and teachers of students with disabilities, and individuals with disabilities (in addition to a myriad of educational and administrative professionals)

(Turnbull & Turnbull, 1998). The I.D.E.A., in conjunction with the Family Educational Rights and Privacy Act (FERPA), addresses issues regarding students' educational records, including access, confidentiality, and privacy.

In ensuring fairness of the process, the school district is required to follow a specific series of steps from the moment that it decides to investigate the potential for a student to qualify for special education. The school district is required to provide to parents a 10 day written notification of any type of MDC and make clear efforts to ensure that parents can attend such meetings. The parents must receive a copy of minutes from the proceedings for all meetings. The school district is required to provide parents with both written and verbal explanations of parents' and students' procedural safeguards under the I.D.E.A., and all written communication must be in the parents' native language. The school district must obtain written informed consent from the parents before initiating any and all components of the NDE/CSE and must obtain written informed consent from the parents again before the child will ever be placed into special education. In other words, providing consent for the evaluation does not mean that parents must, should or otherwise feel obligated, to provide consent for placement into special education. School districts must make efforts to ensure parent participation in the yearly review and development of the IEPs.

Finally, in cases where there is a disagreement between the school district and the parents, the I.D.E.A. provides for an abbreviated court procedure, commonly called due process, that acknowledges the crucial need for timeliness in regards to children's education. These procedures do not necessarily require the involvement of lawyers and are easily scheduled at the parents' and school districts' request.

Disabling Conditions of P.L. 94-142

P.L. 94-142 originally classified 11 handicapping conditions to qualify a child to receive special education and related services. It is crucial to note that the only way children would qualify, even if they have such a condition, is if this disability adversely affects educational performance. In the 1990 amendments to the newly named I.D.E.A., two more disability categories, autism and traumatic brain injury, were added to the previous list of 11 conditions which entitled a child to receive special education and related services. Table 1 outlines the federal classifications of the 13 identified educational disabilities and their federal definitions. A category's inclusion in the list of disability conditions is a

TABLE 1. Federal Classifications of Educational Disabilities (34 C.F.R. § 300.7)

Condition	Definition
Autism	Significant impairment affecting verbal and nonverbal communication and social interaction, generally evident before age 3
Deaf-blindness	Combination of hearing and visual impairments causing severe communication and other developmental and educational needs
Deafness	Severe hearing impairment in processing linguistic information through hearing
Developmental Delay	Expands age range from 3 through 9, significant delays in physical, cognitive, communication, social/emotional, or adaptive development
Emotional Disturbance	An inability to learn; build or maintain satisfactory, interpersonal relationships; inappropriate behavior or feelings; pervasive mood of unhappiness or depression, over a long period and to a marked degree.
Hearing Impairment	Impairment in hearing, whether permanent or fluctuating
Mental Retardation	I.Q. lower than 70; significant difficulty in Adaptive Behavior
Multiple Disability	Concomitant impairments (e.g., mental retardation-blindness) the combination of which causes severe educational needs
Orthopedic Impairment	Severe orthopedic impairments caused by congenital anomaly or from other causes
Other Health Impairment	Limited strength, vitality or alertness, including a heightened alertness to environmental stimuli, due to chronic or acute health problems such as ADD/ADHD
Specific Learning Disability	Disorder of one or more of basic psychological processes that may manifest itself in imperfect ability to listen, think, speak, read, write, spell, or do math
Speech/Language Impairment	Communication disorder, such as stuttering, impaired articulation or voice impairment
Traumatic Brain Injury	Acquired injury to the brain caused by an external physical force, resulting in total or partial functional disability or psychosocial impairment
Visual Impairment/ Blindness	Impairment in vision, even with correction. Partial sight and blindness

Source: Adapted from *"Advocating in schools for children with disabilities: What's new with IDEA?"* By S. J. Altshuler & S. Kopels, 2003, *Social Work, 48,* 320-329.

necessary precursor to ensuring that children with that disability receive appropriate services for their needs. It is important to note that children who are considered as having a disability, but not one that is recognized under the I.D.E.A., have no entitlement to special education and related services as defined by the I.D.E.A. The 1999 amendments further defined some of the 13 conditions to include a wider range of children who are now eligible to qualify for services (Altshuler & Kopels, 2003). The categories of learning disabilities, emotional disturbance and Attention Deficit Disorder will be discussed individually, to provide further explanation of these conditions.

Learning disability: The most frequently labeled disability under the I.D.E.A. is a learning disability, defined as a student demonstrating a significant discrepancy between ability and achievement. Ability is usually measured through I.Q. tests, and is often called the student's ability index or SAI. To qualify as having a learning disability, the student must first demonstrate an SAI that is within the normal range, e.g., no more than 2 standard deviations from the mean. For example, a score of 100 on many I.Q. tests is considered the mean, or the average, score. Thus, for students to begin to qualify for special education services under the I.D.E.A., they must have an S.A.I. score no lower than 80 (if students score higher than 120, while considered gifted, they still may be eligible for learning disability special education services). Once students are assessed to have an intelligence level within the normal range, their achievement must be demonstrated as significantly lower than the mean. That is, students must have scores at least 2 standard deviations below the mean (usually determined by age) of the relevant achievement test. For example, let's say that Kevin, age 10.5, has an S.A.I. of 107, and has been assessed to be reading at the 7.2 level. Because Kevin is reading at 3.3 years lower than his chronological age (10.5 − 7.2 = 3.3), he would be able to qualify for special educational services in reading, under the I.D.E.A. And, indeed, the label requires an additional specification that indicates for which subject (reading, math, written language, etc.) or subjects the student actually qualifies.

Serious Emotional Disturbance/Emotional Disability: This disability is defined having an inability to learn not based on intellectual, sensory or health factors; an inability to establish satisfactory interpersonal relationships with peers and teachers; and inappropriate behaviors or feelings (Knoblauch & Sorenson, 1998). These conditions must be displayed over a long period of time, to a marked degree, such that it adversely affects a child's educational performance (Dupper, 2003). The federal definition excludes the socially-maladjusted, which has created tremendous debates about to whom this is specifically referring. Youth commonly referred to as juvenile delinquents, and indeed chronically truant youth may be classified as socially maladjusted, thereby excluding them from benefiting from special educational services under the I.D.E.A.

Attention Deficit Disorder/Attention Deficit Hyperactivity Disorder (ADD/ADHD): Until 1999, a child with ADD or ADHD did not fall under any of the 13 eligibility categories. Typically, because school districts were not obligated by law to do so, either they would not provide special educational services at all, or they would inappropriately categorize these children as having an emotional disturbance or learning impairment. In some cases, the school district provided children with ADD or ADHD reasonable accommodation plans under Section 504 of the Rehabilitation Act of 1973, but by and large, the special needs of most of these children were not addressed by the public school system (Altshuler & Kopels, 2003).

However, in 1999, children with ADD or ADHD were allowed to be included in the category of other health impairment if their educational performance is hampered by their attention difficulties (Underwood & Kopels, 2004). A child who has ADD or ADHD which adversely affects school performance is now considered to be a child with a disability under I.D.E.A. and entitled to special education and related services.

CONCLUSION

Social workers should be aware of the changing legal rights and protections children and families have regarding education, in order to provide strong advocacy for clients. Because P.L. 94-142 is amended periodically, it is also imperative that all social workers stay abreast of such changes. Probably the most important lesson for social workers is that parents need a supportive advocate at MDCs and any interactional meetings with educational systems.

Attending and participating in I.E.P. meetings at the local school are often unpleasant experiences for parents, especially when they perceive a lack of receptivity to their input and ideas (Hurd & Edwards, 1995; Outland-Mitchell & Anderson, 1992). Armed with knowledge of legal protections, however, social workers and parents can attend these meetings together. Social workers as knowledgeable advocates for parents are in a better position to ensure that parents' voices are heard during such meetings.

All social workers must ensure that parental input is both solicited and received by the school districts when determining a child's eligibility status. Implicit in this imperative is the importance of recognizing the expanded definition of who the parent actually is. Social workers must ensure that the important care givers in children's lives, their parents, grandparents, step-parents, foster parents, are now included in the entire assessment and decision-making process of their children's education (Altshuler & Kopels, 2003). Social workers can provide invaluable support and advocacy to traditionally marginalized clients, including children with disabilities and their families. Social workers encounter such families through health care, mental health and child welfare settings, but do not usually inquire about educational needs of the children. Social workers should ensure that all parental care givers are aware of their rights and the school's responsibilities, and should be prepared to assist them in obtaining needed educational services for their children.

REFERENCES

Allen-Meares, P., Washington, R. O., & Welsh, B. L. (2000). *Social work services in schools* (3rd Ed.). Boston, MA: Allyn & Bacon.

Altshuler, S. J., & Kopels, S. (2003). Advocating in schools for children with disabilities: What's new with IDEA? *Social Work, 48*, 320-329.

Dupper, D. R. (2003). *School social work: Skills and interventions for effective practice.* New Jersey: John H. Wiley & Sons.

Knoblauch, B., & Sorenson, B. (1998). *IDEA's definition of disabilities.* ERIC Document Reproduction Service No. ED429396. Reston, VA: ERIC Clearinghouse on Disabilities and Gifted Education.

To assure the free and appropriate education of all children with disabilities. Twentieth annual report to Congress on the implementation of the Individuals with Disabilities Act (1998). U.S. Department of Education, Office of Special Education Programs. Washington, DC: Author.

Turnbull, H. R., & Turnbull, A. P. (1998). *Free appropriate public education: The law and children with disabilities* (3rd Ed.). Denver: Love Publishing.

Underwood, D. J., & Kopels, S. (2004). Complaints filed against schools by parents of children with AD/HD: Implications for school social work practice. *Children & Schools, 26*, 221-233.

doi:10.1300/J198v06n01_02

MiCASSA–
My Home

Reiko Hayashi

SUMMARY. This article will introduce people with disabilities as change agents who affect policy enactments and implementation in this country. It will begin with a brief description of a bill (H.R. 2032/S.971), the Medicaid Community Attendant Services and Supports Act (MiCASSA). That will be followed by the grassroots history of the disability-rights movement since the 1960s and the independent living philosophy that was born in the movement and underlies the development of MiCASSA. The contributions to the MiCASSA bill by Section 504 of the Rehabilitation Act, the Americans With Disabilities Act, and the Supreme Court's Olmstead Decision will be presented. Finally, MiCASSA's implications to both social work education and practice will be discussed. doi:10.1300/J198v06n01_03 *[Article copies available for a fee from The Haworth Document Delivery Service: 1-800-HAWORTH. E-mail address: <docdelivery@haworth press.com> Website: <http://www.HaworthPress.com> © 2007 by The Haworth Press, Inc. All rights reserved.]*

KEYWORDS. MiCASSA, disability rights movement, independent living, ADA, Olmstead

---

Reiko Hayashi, PhD, MSW, is Associate Professor, College of Social Work, University of Utah, 395 South 1500 East Room 207, Salt Lake City, UT 84112-0260 (E-mail: Reiko.Hayashi@socwk.utah.edu).

[Haworth co-indexing entry note]: "MiCASSA–My Home." Hayashi, Reiko. Co-published simultaneously in *Journal of Social Work in Disability & Rehabilitation* (The Haworth Press, Inc.) Vol. 6, No. 1/2, 2007, pp. 35-52; and: *Disability and Social Work Education: Practice and Policy Issues* (ed: Francis K. O. Yuen, Carol B. Cohen, and Kristine Tower) The Haworth Press, Inc., 2007, pp. 35-52. Single or multiple copies of this article are available for a fee from The Haworth Document Delivery Service [1-800-HAWORTH, 9:00 a.m. - 5:00 p.m. (EST). E-mail address: docdelivery@haworthpress.com].

Available online at http://jswdr.haworthpress.com
© 2007 by The Haworth Press, Inc. All rights reserved.
doi:10.1300/J198v06n01_03

INTRODUCTION

This article will introduce the Medicaid Community Attendant Services and Supports Act (MiCASSA). If passed, this bill (H.R. 2032/S. 971) will enable people with disabilities who reside in nursing homes to move to community settings. Because Medicaid funding for long-term care favors institutionalization over community-based care, many disabled Medicaid recipients live in nursing homes even though they would prefer to live in their own homes in the community (HCFA, 2000a). MiCASSA will allow Medicaid money presently paid for nursing-home care to move with the recipient when she or he chooses to live in a community setting.

The intention of this article is not solely to examine MiCASSA as a long-term care policy that affects the lives of people with disabilities per se, but to discuss the civil-rights issues on which disability rights advocates have been working for years. Although social workers and other human services personnel provide services defined by legislation and social policies, they often are unaware of the political history of those policies. Perhaps their 19th century origins as charity workers (Abramovitz, 1998; Margolin, 1997) continues to affect social workers' perceptions of people with disabilities, and many continue to view disability issues from a perspective of charity rather than civil-rights.

People with disabilities as change agents who affect policy enactments and implementation in this country will be introduced. It will start with a brief description of MiCASSA, followed by the grassroots history of the disability-rights movement since the 1960s and the independent living philosophy that was born in the movement and underlies the development of MiCASSA. The contributions to the MiCASSA bill by Section 504 of the Rehabilitation Act, the Americans With Disabilities Act, and the Supreme Court's Olmstead Decision will be discussed. Finally, MiCASSA's implications to both social work education and practice will be presented.

WHAT IS MICASSA?

Currently, people eligible for Medicaid and in need of personal care services often receive those services in nursing homes even though they would prefer to live in community settings. Because Medicaid requires states to pay for nursing-home services while community-based care remains an option, nursing homes continue to be the service of choice.

States can apply for Home- and Community-Based Services (HCBS) waivers (1915(c)) to obtain federal Medicaid matching funds to create and provide long-term care services to clients in the community settings (NASMD, 2002). But the HCBS programs vary among states in both quality and scope, and the funding is more limited than funding for nursing-home care (Fox-Grage, Folkemer, & Lewis, 2003). In 2002, 70% of Medicaid's long-term care funds–$57 billion–supported institutional care (Eiken, 2003).

The MiCASSA bill (H.R. 2032/S. 971) would amend Medicaid to provide individuals eligible for nursing-home services the option to live in a community setting and receive in-home attendant services and support. Medicaid institutional-care funds would move with clients who move from an institution to a community setting. Further, MiCASSA requires that services be provided in the most integrated setting appropriate to the needs of the individual. To accomplish this, clients would be given a choice of various service delivery models (e.g., self-directed or case-managed), compensation would be provided for the transition costs of their move from a nursing home to a community setting, and service quality would be assured by promoting client control and satisfaction. If MiCASSA passes, services provided by HCBS programs will be expanded, reducing unwanted institutionalization. States currently implementing successful HCBS programs could expand services and modify the infrastructures they already have in place.

DISABILITY RIGHTS MOVEMENT

Let's examine the historical events that have occurred since the 1960s, events that provide the background for MiCASSA. The civil rights and feminist movements of the 1960s helped change societal norms and improve the treatment of people of color and women. While efforts to fully achieve equal rights for people of color and women are ongoing, our society now acknowledges that it is illegal to segregate people of color or deny women access to jobs or education or other opportunities available to men. Although less well known, the modern disability rights movement also began in 1960s. Disability advocates during these 40+ years have been instrumental in the enactment of disability-rights legislation, including the Americans With Disabilities Act (ADA) of 1990 which recognizes the civil rights of people with disabilities. Although many people would still prefer the segregation of people with disabilities and would rather deny people with disabilities access to the opportunities that are available to nondisabled people, we now see students with disabilities rolling on college campuses and many business establishments accommodating disabled customers.

In 1962 Ed Roberts, a quadriplegic young man and ventilator user was accepted to the University of California, Berkeley. Not being able to accommodate him and his iron lung in a dorm, the university housed him in a room at Cowell Hospital, the on-campus student health center. Within the next few years a dozen other students with disabilities joined him at Cowell. They created a group known as the Rolling Quads that worked to make the campus and the city of Berkeley accessible. In 1972, the Rolling Quads founded the first center for independent living in Berkeley, and Roberts became the director of the center (Brown, 2000; Shapiro, 1993, pp. 41-73).

In Denver, Colorado, a group of young adult former residents of a nursing home founded the second independent living center, Atlantis, in 1975. They realized that no amount of outings to concerts or bingo games could fulfill their lives. They wanted to live in their own apartments in the community and create self-determined lifestyles with the freedom to choose their own food, direct their own care, and determine their own priorities (Atlantis, 1998). During the next thirty years, centers for independent living arose in every state in the United States and others were launched abroad. Currently there are about 400 centers for independent living in the U.S. that are managed by people with disabilities and provide advocacy work as well as social services to support disabled people living in the community (DeJong, Batavia, & McKnew, 1992; Lifchez, 1979).

In 1977, a memorable event occurred in the history of disability rights. Although President Nixon had signed the Rehabilitation Act of 1973, and Section 504 prohibited organizations that receive federal funds from discriminating against people on the basis of disability, the Department of Health Education and Welfare (HEW) refused to issue regulations to implement the law, expressing concerns about costs and administrative annoyance. In 1977, disability advocates found that HEW Secretary Joseph Califano of the new Carter administration was also unwilling to issue regulations. Demanding the implementation of the Section 504, more than 150 disability advocates took over the federal building in San Francisco and staged a sit-in for 25 days. The protest gained community support, the mayor of San Francisco ordered law enforcement personnel to leave them alone, and the Black Panthers and Gray Panthers brought in food. After 25 days, Secretary Calfano signed the regulations. Section 504 of the Rehabilitation Act is regarded as the precursor of the Americans With Disabilities Act (ADA), and the successful peaceful protest that led to its implementation nurtured a sense of pride and solidarity in the disability community (Brown, 2000; Shapiro, 1993, pp. 55-73).

INDEPENDENT LIVING PHILOSOPHY

The independent living philosophy was born in the disability rights movement. Three essential premises provide the scaffolding for the independent living philosophy: (1) each individual is different and unique; (2) people with disabilities are the most knowledgeable experts about their own needs and issues; and (3) programs serving disabled people should be designed to serve all disability groups. The first premise reminds us that each person with a disability, like each person without a disability, is unique and should not be labeled or categorized by that disability. The second premise recognizes and promotes the empowerment and self-determination of people with disabilities, and encourages peer support and consumer control of services. The third premise has led to the concept of cross-disability. Given that all people with disabilities are oppressed, independent living programs need to be designed to empower and serve all people regardless of types of disabilities and ensure equal social, cultural, economic, and political opportunities for all (Brown, 2000).

ADAPT

As the independent living philosophy and practice spread to many areas of the country, a group of people with disabilities started its national campaign for access to public transit in 1983. They claimed that without accessible public transit, they were confined to their residences, and they recognized this as an act of discrimination. Calling themselves "American Disabled for Accessible Public Transit" (ADAPT), they employed civil disobedience and other non-violent direct action tactics, including blocking buses in cities across the United States, to dramatize their demand for equal access to public transit (ADAPT, 1997).

While continuing to work on the public transit issue ADAPT took the de-institutionalization of people with disabilities as the next agenda. As described previously, many people with disabilities who needed personal care services had been placed in nursing homes even though they desired to live in their own homes with some support from personal attendants. In 1990 ADAPT renamed themselves as "American Disabled for Attendant Programs Today" and directed their activism on the reallocation of the Medicaid dollars from institutional programs to consumer controlled community based programs (ADAPT, 1997).

THE AMERICANS WITH DISABILITIES ACT

In 1990, another historically significant year for the disability rights community, the U.S. Congress enacted the Americans With Disabilities Act (ADA), which recognized civil rights for people with disabilities. The goals of the ADA include ensuring equality of opportunity, full participation, independent living, and economic self-sufficiency for people with disabilities. Individualization, meaningful opportunity, inclusion, and empowerment are key concepts articulated in the ADA (Burgdorf, 1991; Silverstein, 2003). Title I addresses the issue of employment discrimination. Title II prohibits public entities from discriminating against disabled people and requires that state and local governments give them an equal opportunity to benefit from all of their programs, services, and activities. Title III makes discrimination against disabled people illegal in public accommodations and in commercial facilities. Title IV mandates the establishment of telecommunication's relay services (U.S. Department of Justice, 2002).

Title II is further described here because it is the basis of the Olmstead decision, introduced later in this article, which strengthens MiCASSA. Congress described the isolation and segregation of people with disabilities as a serious and pervasive form of discrimination. Title II denotes that no qualified individual with a disability shall, "by reason of such disability," be excluded from participation in, or be denied the benefits of, a public entity's services, programs, or activities. Congress ordered the Attorney General to issue regulations to prohibit discrimination based on Title II. The regulations include the "integration regulation" which requires public entities to administer programs in the most integrated setting appropriate to the needs of qualified individuals with disabilities. They also include a "reasonable-modifications regulation" which requires public entities to make reasonable modifications to avoid discrimination on the basis of disability (Legal Information Institute, 1999).

Undergirding the enactment of the ADA was, of course, many years of advocacy work by people like Justin Dart and others in the disability rights movement. Justin Dart, who is recognized as the father of ADA, was photographed in July of 1990 with other advocates on the White House lawn as President George H. Bush signed the ADA into law (Disability History Museum, 2004).

NOT DEAD YET

The 1990s was also the decade when the media often focused on the issue of doctor-assisted suicide of people with disabilities. The concept of a "life worse than death" was emphasized as Dr. Jack Kevorkian challenged the judicial system and killed more than 130 people with disabilities, most of whom were not terminally ill (Humphry, 2003). To counter public acquiescence to doctor-assisted suicide for people with disabilities, Not Dead Yet, an organization of people with disabilities was founded in 1996. The founder of the organization, Diane Coleman (1999), proclaimed:

> [T]he idea that people with disabilities are not worthy of society's acceptance or resources is not new. We see this form of hatred throughout history, often masked as benevolence. But for the first time in history, people with disabilities are organizing our community to fight back, to demand the equal protection of the law.

When a nondisabled person asks for an assistance to commit suicide, it is generally taken as a cry for help. Concerned people try to help and he or she is referred to counseling. But when a disabled person does the same thing, that "cry for help" is misinterpreted and the "wish" may well be granted.

The book "No Pity" (Shapiro, 1993) introduces Larry James McAfee and his ordeal. Larry McAffee became quadriplegic and a respirator user as a result of a motorcycle accident in Georgia. Bounced from one nursing home to another because no institution in Georgia wanted to keep him due to the low Medicaid reimbursement rate, he ended up languishing in the ICU ward of a hospital for months. Finally, he requested a court order for doctor-assisted suicide. He told the judge that his life as a quadriplegic had been intolerable.

Fortunately, by the time the judge decided to grant his wish (after praising him for his bravery and receiving hugs and thanks from Larry's mother for showing such compassion), Larry had already moved to a nursing home in Alabama. And at this point he was in no hurry to return to Georgia to die because disability advocates there had shown him life's possibilities. After learning to use a power wheelchair and a computer with his breath, he left the nursing home to live in an apartment with attendant care.

When Larry McAffee requested doctor-assisted suicide, no one tested him for depression or examined his living environment. Had they done so, they would have understood that Larry was depressed because his quality of life was diminished by the poor treatment he received in nursing homes. Regarded with indifference and suffering from neglect, he had been wasting away in his bed, with little opportunity to doing anything more than gaze at the ceiling (Shapiro, 1993, pp 258-288).

Not Dead Yet (2002) argued that people have the right to refuse unwanted treatment, and that suicide is not illegal. Furthermore, they contended that making doctor-assisted suicide a public policy that singles out individuals for legalized killing based on health status violates the Americans With Disabilities Act (Coleman, 2000).

In 1999, Dr. Jack Kevorkian was sentenced to 10-25 years for the second-degree murder of Thomas Youk. Although Not Dead Yet consider his sentence as justice served, one year later the Gleitsman Foundation awarded Kevorkian its Citizen Activist Award for his humanitarian work. Co-recipient of the award was Bryan Stevenson, an attorney and anti-death penalty activist from Alabama. The awards committee included Marian Wright Edelman of the Children's Defense Fund, Stanley Sheinbaum of Human Rights Watch, feminist Gloria Steinem, and Morris Dees of the Southern Poverty Law Center (Reynolds, 2000). It was disheartening for people with disabilities to learn that even prominent human rights advocates could not see that presenting such an award to Dr. Kevorkian was tacit rejection of the fundamental right to live for people with disabilities. As Not Dead Yet continues to fight for the right to live for people with disabilities, ADAPT continues to fight for "right to choose" for people with disabilities via the establishment of MiCASSA.

THE MICASSA BILL

In 1997, Representative Newt Gingrich (R-GA) introduced the original MiCASA bill to Congress. This was a direct result of ADAPT's strategy. When Newt Gingrich became the Speaker of the House after the Republicans gained control of the House for the first time in 40 years, ADAPT targeted Gingrich for their lobbying efforts. ADAPT members visited Gingrich at his home and offices in Georgia and Washington, DC, and demanded that he introduce a bill that would reform Medicaid so that unnecessary institutionalization of people with disabilities would be avoided. When he traveled to other cities, ADAPT branches in those cities also showed up at his events. When he finally agreed to work on the bill, ADAPT began educating Gingrich and his staff about the issue. In 1997, three hundred ADAPT members showed up at the Capitol and demanded that the bill be introduced. Gingrich agreed to draft the language. His staff and ADAPT leadership immediately worked on the language in the basement of the House Office building for three hours and drafted House Bill 2020. Then Gingrich introduced the original MiCASSA bill to Congress (Kafka, 2003).

THE OLMSTEAD DECISION

In 1999, the U.S. Supreme Court ruled in the case of *Olmstead vs. L. C. and E.W.* The Olmstead decision interpreted Title II of the ADA, declaring that unnecessary institutionalization of individuals with disabilities is discrimination and that the state must provide services in the most integrated setting appropriate to individual clients (Silverstein, 2003; CMS, 2002).

Plaintiffs L.C. and E.W. were people with mental retardation and psychiatric disabilities. Both were voluntarily admitted to a Georgia hospital's psychiatric unit. Although their doctors eventually evaluated them and agreed that they could be cared for in a community-based program, they continued to be housed in the hospital. L.C. filed suit against the state of Georgia, contending that it violated Title II in failing to place her in a community-based program. E.W. joined the suit, stating an identical accusation (Legal Information Institute, 1999).

The State argued that inadequate funding, not discrimination, was the cause of their confinement to the hospital. But the District Court rejected the State's argument and concluded that unnecessary institutionalization constitutes discrimination, which cannot be justified by a lack of funding (Legal Information Institute, 1999). The Supreme Court upheld the decision of the lower court. Justice Ginsburg delivered the opinion of the court:

> Under Title II of the ADA states are required to place people with mental disabilities in community settings rather than in institutions when the State's treatment professionals have determined that community placement is appropriate, the transfer from institutional care to a less restrictive setting is not opposed by the affected individual,

and the placement can be reasonably accommodated, taking into account the resources available to the State and the needs of others with mental disabilities. (National Center for An Accessible Society, 1999)

The Olmstead decision stresses that people with disabilities should not be forced to relinquish their civil right to live in the community in order to receive medical services (Silverstein, 2003). It challenges Federal, state, and local governments to develop and administer their services "in the most integrated setting appropriate to the needs of qualified individuals with disabilities." These governmental institutions have been challenged to develop more opportunities for individuals with disabilities through more accessible systems of community-based services. Although the plaintiffs of this case were people with mental retardation and psychiatric disabilities, the Olmstead decision covers all people with disabilities, including the elderly. Although applications of the ADA and the Olmstead decision are not limited to programs funded by Medicaid, Medicaid recipients are among the most affected.

To comply with the Olmstead decision, the Center for Medicare and Medicaid Services (CMS) has encouraged state governors and state Medicaid directors to develop community-based services. CMS offers system-change grants to states to develop systems to move nursing-home residents to community settings. States are required to do self-evaluations to ensure that their policies, practices, and procedures promote community-based services (Shalala, 2000; Westmoreland, 2000a, 2000b, 2000c, 2001a, 2001b).

SPONSORS AND SUPPORTERS

Encouraged by the Olmstead decision, ADAPT and other disability advocates stepped up their lobbying efforts. In 2001, Senators Harkin (D-IA), Kennedy (D-MA), Clinton (D-NY), Biden (D-DE), and Specter (R-PA) co-sponsored the MiCASSA bill to the Senate. In 2002, Representatives Davis (D-IL) and Shimkus (R-IL) reintroduced the bill in the House. As of May 2004, the bill has 17 co-sponsors in the Senate and 101 co-sponsors in the House.

MiCASSA is also gaining support from many professional and advocacy organizations. As of January 2004, 92 national organizations support the bill, including the American Association on Mental Retardation, American Geriatrics Society, American Rehabilitation Counseling Association, Brain Injury Association, Families USA, NAACP, National

Association of Area Agencies on Aging, National Council on the Aging, National Council on Independent Living, National Spinal Cord Injury Association, NOW, Service Employees International Union, and US Conference of Mayors. Further, hundreds of local- and state-level organizations support the bill. Yet among social-work institutions, only the Texas NASW chapter officially supports MiCASSA (ADAPT, 2004). Not surprisingly, the American Health Care Association–the association of the nursing-home industry–opposes the bill (AHCA, 2003).

COST OF LONG-TERM CARE AND THE AGING POPULATION

After the Olmstead decision compelled state governments to develop community-based long-term care programs, it soon became clear that community-based services can cost less than the institutional care (National Association of state Medicaid Directors, 2004). Figure 1 shows Medicaid nursing-home expenditures as a percentage of the total US nursing-home care costs in 1968 and 1998 (HCFA, 2000b). Medicaid spending includes state and federal shares. In 1968, less than one fourth of the nursing-home care expenditure was borne by Medicaid. Thirty years later, the share had increased to 46%. Furthermore, the total spending on nursing-home care was only $2.9 billion in 1968. In 1998, it was $87.8 billion. Not only did Medicaid's share of nursing-home costs increase, but also the dollar amount increased dramatically as well.

FIGURE 1. Medicaid Nursing Home Expenditures as a Percent of Total U.S. Nursing Home Care Expenditures, Calendar Years 1968 and 1998

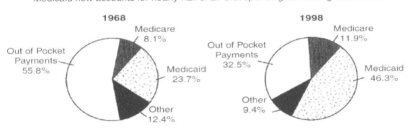

Medicaid now accounts for nearly half of all U.S. spending on nursing home care.

Note: Medicaid spending includes the state and federal shares. Total U.S. spending on nursing home care was $87.8 billion in 1998 compared to $2.9 billion in 1968. The 1998 "other" expenditures primarily consists of private health insurance and Veteran's Administration spending. The 1968 "other" consisted largely of non-Medicaid general funds from state/local and federal governments. Percentages may not sum to 100 due to rounding.

Source: HCFA/Office of the Actuary, National Health Statistics Group.

People are living longer, and baby-boomers are getting old. It is inevitable that self-paying nursing-home residents will eventually use up their assets and become Medicaid recipients. As a result, the government share of long-term care expenditures is expected to increase correlatively. Therefore, community-based services for long-term care will be a cost-saving alternative for states.

ROLES OF SOCIAL WORKERS
IN LIVES OF PEOPLE WITH DISABILITIES

The preceding brief history of the disability civil rights movement and its link to the MiCASSA bill leads us to the role of social work in the lives of people with disabilities and how social workers can contribute to the establishment and execution of MiCASSA.

Many people with disabilities have contact with social workers in their lives. Social workers may visit disabled people to assess eligibility for HCBS waiver programs. Social workers may arrange various community services for disabled people. And social workers may work in nursing homes and create a discharge plans for disabled residents. Unfortunately, social workers are generally not highly regarded by disability advocates. Instead, they are considered an annoyance at best, but a necessary one since they are in charge of evaluations that will determine needed services. At worst, social workers are seen as prison guards of concentration camps and thieves of human dignity with power over people with disabilities.

A former nursing-home resident and wheelchair user in her late thirties recalls her life in an institution and the social workers she encountered.

> [I] had no choice at all. They–social workers and nursing staff–made all choices. They run your life. You do it the way they want you to do it. They schedule the day. They decide what's good behavior, what's bad behavior. They decide if you are overweight or not. They put you on a diet without your consent. If they decide you have bad behavior, depending on the "bad behavior" you either get chastised about it or have your activities restricted. I was always chastised for standing up for myself. I had feelings of frustration and anger. They treated me like a kid. I lost my dignity and freedom. They were taken. They make you live by their rules, not yours. It's like being a herd of cattle. It's totally demoralizing.

The cruelest thing was that they told me that I would never leave the nursing home. My social worker told me, 'You must stay here for the rest of your life.' I said, 'But you are my social worker, you have to help me get out of here.' She said, 'All staff think that you should stay here, and I agree with them.' She was supposed to be my social worker, but she worked for the nursing home, not for me. They said that to lots of people . . . (Hayashi, 2005, p. 5)

Many people with disabilities perceive social workers and case-managers as agents of control. From their standpoint, social workers have the attitude that they know what is better for disabled people than do the people themselves, and consequently social workers try to control their lives. For those people with disabilities, social workers are representatives of the system that oppresses them (Hayashi & Rousculp, 2004).

Margolin (1997) describes a discordant juxtaposition of social-work theory and practice which may contribute to the existing high level of burnout in the profession. Although social workers often talk about client empowerment and self-determination, in practice they encourage client conformity and oppose client resistance. Unlike earlier social-work orthodoxy that viewed clients as inferior and helpless, current social-work doctrine promotes empathy, cultural sensitivity, and client empowerment. It recognizes that problems manifested in clients often are the result of outside causes, including "institutionalized oppression" and a "white middle-class power structure." Nevertheless, the old methods of social-work intervention have remained largely unchanged. The focus of change has not been on institutional structure but on the client. The social-work profession has instinctively ignored this contradiction in order to persist as an occupation (Margolin, 1997).

Rose (2000) also argues that while the social-work profession formally promotes a political commitment to social justice and equality, its focus in practice is on human behavioral theories that pathologize individual clients. This practice diverts attention away from the social structures that foster oppression. Social workers have the power to diagnose, interpret, and label a client's behaviors. In stark contrast to written theoretical tenets, they covertly and unknowingly act as agents of social control. While harboring the erroneous belief that these actions are helping their clients, they are instead oppressing their clients while maintaining the status quo.

Thompson (2000) discusses the existence of formal and informal theories of social work practice. Formal practice theories are found in academic literature and publications of professional organizations, and they are taught in social work classrooms. On the other hand, informal practice theories which are not published in official literature constitute the "practice wisdom" of the social work profession. They are "culturally transmitted" to new generations of social workers in agencies and in the field. While formal practice theory, such as empowerment theory, is discussed in classrooms and debated in professional journals, informal practice theory is carried out without discussion in the field. The strong animosity of some people with disabilities against social-work professionals may come from their experience with the "practice wisdom" that views people with disabilities as inferior beings and troublemakers.

IMPLICATIONS FOR SOCIAL WORK EDUCATION

Although social workers have served clients with disabilities for years, disability issues were rarely taught as diversity issues or civil-rights issues in social work classrooms until recently. Instead, the medical model of disability has been and continues to be taught. This approach treats disability as a personal tragedy, something that should be "fixed" by professional intervention (Gilson, 2002; Gilson & Depoy, 2002; Hahn, 1988; Mackelprang & Salsgiver, 1998).

Today, many social work educators who teach diversity courses require their students to reflect on their background (e.g., race, ethnicity, class, gender, sexual orientation) and ponder their feelings about their own identities and how those identities have affected their lives and their perceptions of the world. It is considered important to learn about oneself in order to understand and empathize with clients from various backgrounds (NASW, 2003).

This exercise should also be required regarding disability issues. Nondisabled students need to consider their status in the ableist society where prejudice towards people with disabilities is prevalent. Hahn (1988) discusses two kinds of anxiety–aesthetic and existential–that nondisabled people experience when they encounter a person with a disability. Aesthetic anxiety is aroused when people encounter those who look different and are physically outside the societal norm. In contemporary society where good looks are highly valued, young, beautiful, slim, and able-bodied defines the norm. Since disabilities violate this norm, nondisabled people feel uncomfortable and anxious when they encounter people with disabilities.

Existential anxiety is aroused in people when they are reminded of their own vulnerability to disability. Unlike one's race, a person can change his or her status from able-bodied to disabled overnight by an accident or an illness. Nondisabled people, who rarely consider their vulnerability to disability, feel uncomfortable and anxious when they encounter people with disabilities who remind them of their vulnerability (Hahn, 1988). Nondisabled students need to explore and struggle with their anxieties towards people with disabilities and how societal norms contribute to those feelings. Students with disabilities must consider their own levels of internalized ableism just as those students who are members of other oppressed groups confront internalized oppression that leads to self-devaluation (Freire, 1970).

Social work students also need to learn about the historical segregation of people with disabilities and the social policies that have supported such discriminatory practices. And finally, all social work students should learn about the history of the disability rights movement and its contributions to changes in policy. MiCASSA should be one of those policies introduced in the classroom.

As discussed in the previous section, social work education must acknowledge the disparity between the rhetoric of social work and the realities endured in practice by clients including people with disabilities in the long-term care field (Margolin, 1997; Rose, 2000; Thompson, 2000). Finn and Jacobson (2003) state that although a commitment to institutional change has been promoted in both social work theory and practice in other countries (especially in South America), it has been marginalized in the United States where strategies for personal or interpersonal change tend to overshadow the institutional-change approach. They call for social workers in this country to return to the work of social justice.

The knowledge students' gain in a diversity course about disability issues could be applied to macro social work courses such as those in administration, community organizations, and advocacy to carry out social-justice work. Dickinson (2003) reports that social workers are generally uncomfortable with social action. Social work has been professionalized since the time of Jane Addams and Hull House, and social workers may feel that social actions such as those led by ADAPT are not professional pursuits. Still, social workers and social work students could organize to lobby legislators for MiCASSA and other policies that enhance the civil rights of people with disabilities (Amidei, 1991; Schneider & Lester, 2000). They could also educate Their colleagues about disability issues and promote ways to change the traditionally ableist service-delivery system in long-term care service agencies.

The civil-rights struggle is on-going. It is not just an event in the past that we read about in textbooks. It is happening in the everyday lives of people with disabilities, in social work classrooms, in social service institutions, on the streets, in the courts, and in Congress. Social workers should actively participate in that struggle if we are true to our professional mission of social justice. The MiCASSA legislation presents us with an opportunity for active participation.

REFERENCES

Abramovitz, M. (1988). *Regulating the lives of women: Social welfare policy from colonial times to the present*. Boston, MA: South End Press.

ADAPT (1997). Real homes not nursing homes. Retrieved May 24, 2004 from http://www.adapt.org/back.htm

ADAPT (2004). Current supporters of MiCASSA. Retrieved May 25, 2004 from http://www.adapt.org/casa/supporters.htm

American Health Care Association (AHCA) (2003). Issue Brief: MiCASSA Legislation. Retrieved May 25, 2005 from http://www.ahca.org/brief/ib_micassa.pdf

Amidei, N. (1991). *So you want to make a difference: A key to advocacy*. Washington, DC: Omb Watch.

Atlantis (1998). A history of liberation. Atlantis Independent Living Center. Retrieved May 24, 2004 from http://www.atlantiscom.org/index.html

Brown, S.E. (2000). Freedom of movement: Independent living history and philosophy. Institute on Disability Culture. Retrieved June 24, 2004 from http://www.ilru.org/ilnet/files/bookshelf/freedom

Burgdorf, R. (1991). The Americans With Disabilities Act: Analysis and implications of a second-generation civil rights statute. *Harvard Civil Rights/Civil Liberties Law Review, 26*, 413-522.

Centers for Medicare & Medicaid Services (CMS) (2002). Americans With Disabilities Act/Olmstead Decision. Retrieved May 05, 2004 from http://www.cms.hhs.gov/olmstead/default.asp

Coleman, D. (1999). Not dead yet: The resistance. Retrieved May 24, 2004 from http://www.notdeadyet.org

Coleman, D. (2000). Assisted suicide and disability: Another perspective. *Human Rights*. American Bar Association. Retrieved May 24, 2004 from http://www.abanet.org/irr/hr/winter00humanrights/colemand.html

DeJong, G., Batavia, A., & McKnew, L. (1992). The independent living model of personal assistance in long-term-care policy. *Generations, 16*, 89-95.

Dickinson, J. (2003). Attitudes of social workers in South Carolina toward social action. Paper presented at the 2003 Policy Conference for Social Work Education and Practice.

Disability History Museum (2004). Library collection: Visuals–catalog card. Retrieved May 15, 2004 from http://www.disabilitymuseum.org/lib/stills/599card.htm

Eiken, S. (2003). Follow the money: Trends in state spending. Thomson Medstat. Retrieved May 28, 2004 from http://www.nasua.org/hcbsppt/Session%201-G%20Steve%20Eiken.ppt

Finn, J.L., & Jacobson, M. (2003). Just practice: Steps toward a new social work paradigm. *Journal of Social Work Education, 39*(1), 57-78.

Fox-Grage, W., Folkemer, D., & Lewis, J. (2003). The states' response to the Olmstead decision: How are states complying? National Conference of State Legislatures. Retrieved June 24, 2004 from http://www.ncsl.org/programs/health/forum/olms report.htm

Freire, P (1970). Pedagogy of the oppressed. New York: Continuum.

Gilson, S.F. (Ed.) (2002). *Integrating disability content in social work education.* Alexandria, VI: Council on Social Work Education.

Gilson, S.F., & Depoy E. (2002). Theoretical approaches to disability content in social work education. *Journal of Social Work Education, 38*(1), 153-165.

Hahn, H. (1988). The politics of physical differences: Disability and discrimination. *Journal of Social Issues, 44*(1), 39-47.

Hayashi, R. (2005). The environment of disability today: A nursing home is not a home. In G. May & M. Raske (Eds.) *Ending disability discrimination: Strategies for social workers.* (pp. 45-71). Boston, MA: Allyn and Bacon.

Hayashi, R., & Rousculp, T. (2004). The "Our Homes, Not Nursing Homes" project: Lives of people with disabilities in nursing homes. *Journal of Social Work in Disability & Rehabilitation, 3*(2), 57-70.

Health Care Financing Administration (HCFA) (2000a). Medicaid spending for institutional long-term care and home and community care (Figure 4.5). A profile of Medicaid: Chart book 2000. U.S. Department Of Health and Human Services. Retrieved May 24, 2004 from http://cms.hhs.gov/charts/medicaid/2tchartbk.pdf

Health Care Financing Administration (HCFA) (2000b). Medicaid nursing home expenditures as a percent of total U.S. nursing home care expenditures, Calendar Years 1968 and 1998 (Figure 4.4). A profile of Medicaid: Chart book 2000. U.S. Department Of Health and Human Services. Retrieved May 24, 2004 from http://cms. hhs.gov/charts/medicaid/2tchartbk.pdf

Humphry, D. (2003). Prisoner of conscience: Dr. Jack Kevorkian, Prisoner #284797– Martyr to the cause of the right to choose to die. Euthanasia Research and Guidance Organization. Retrieved May 24, 2004 from http://www.finalexit.org/drkframe.html

Kafka, B. (2003). Personal communication. Chair of ADAPT.

Legal Information Institute (1999). OLMSTEAD V. L. C. (98-536) 527 U.S. 581. Supreme Court Collection. Cornell Law School. Retrieved May 24, 2004 from http:// supct.law.cornell.edu/supct/html/98-536.ZS.html

Lifchez, R. (1979). *Design for independent living.* Berkeley: University of California Press.

Mackelprang, R. W., & Salsgiver, R. O. (1998). *Disability: A diversity model approach in human service practice.* Pacific Grove, CA: Brooks/Cole Publishing Company.

Margolin, L. (1997). *Under the cover of kindness: The intervention of social work.* Charlottesville & London: University Press of Virginia.

National Association of State Medicaid Directors (NASMD) (2002). Medicaid waivers. Retrieved June 24, 2004 from http://www.nasmd.org/waivers/waivers.htm

National Association of Social Workers (NASW) (2003). Cultural competence in the social work profession.*Social Work Speaks*, 71-74. Retrieved May 15, 2004. http:// www.socialworkers.org/da/da2005/documents/cultcompswprof.pdf

National Center for an Accessible Society (1999). Supreme Court upholds ADA 'Integration Mandate' in *Olmstead* decision. Retrieved May 24, 2004 from http://www. accessiblesociety.org/topics/ada/olmsteadoverview.htm

Not Dead Yet (2002). Not dead yet: The resistance. Retrieved May 25, 2004 from http://www.notdeadyet.org

Reynolds, D. (2000). Controversy stirred up over Kevorkian award. *Inclusion Daily Express*, April 10, 2000. Retrieved May 24, 2004 from http://www.inclusiondaily.com/news/advocacy/kevorkian.htm#041100

Rose, S.M. (2000). Reflections on empowerment-based practice. *Social Work 45*(5), 403-412.

Schneider, R., & Lester, L. (2000). *Social work advocacy: A new framework for action.* Boston: Wadsworth Publishing.

Shalala, D.E. (2000). HHS Secretary's Letter to Governors on Olmstead Decision. Retrieved May 25, 2004 from http://www.cms.hhs.gov/states/letters/smd1140b.asp

Shapiro, J.P. (1993). *No pity: People with disabilities forging a new civil rights movement.* New York, NY: Times Books.

Silverstein, R. (2003). Olmstead vs. L.C.–*An Overview and Description of the U.S. Supreme Court Decision.* Center for the Study and Advancement of Disability Policy (CSADP). Retrieved May 24, 2004 from http://www.pacer.org/tatra/olmstead_LC.htm

Thompson, N. (2000). *Theory and practice in human services.* Buckingham: Open University Press.

U.S. Department of Justice (2002). Public Law 101-36: Americans With Disabilities Act of 1990. Retrieved May 24, 2004 from http://www.usdoj.gov/crt/ada/pubs/ada.txt

Westmoreland, T.M. (2000a). Nursing home transition grant 2000–May 31, 2000 ADA/Olmstead Decision State Medicaid Director Letters. Retrieved May 25, 2004 from http://www.cms.hhs.gov/olmstead/smdltrs.asp

Westmoreland, T.M. (2000b). Olmstead update No.2 Questions and answers–July 25, 2000. ADA/Olmstead Decision State Medicaid Director Letters. Retrieved May 25, 2004 from http://www.cms.hhs.gov/olmstead/smdltrs.asp

Westmoreland, T.M. (2000c). Olmstead update No. 3 Update–July 25, 2000. ADA/Olmstead Decision State Medicaid Director Letters. Retrieved May 25, 2004 from http://www.cms.hhs.gov/olmstead/smdltrs.asp

Westmoreland, T.M. (2001a). Olmstead update No. 4 Update–January 10, 2001 ADA/Olmstead Decision State Medicaid Director Letters. Retrieved May 25, 2004 from http://www.cms.hhs.gov/olmstead/smdltrs.asp

Westmoreland, T.M. (2001b). Olmstead update No. 5 New tools for states–January 10, 2001 ADA/Olmstead Decision State Medicaid Director Letters. Retrieved May 25, 2004 from http://www.cms.hhs.gov/olmstead/smdltrs.asp

doi:10.1300/J198v06n01_03

Resources Ancillary Services and Classroom Instruction: Thoughts of a Deaf-Blind Social Work Student and Her Teacher

Teresa V. Mason
Ashleigh Smith

SUMMARY. This article is the story of a social work instructor and her deaf-blind student. The chapter includes: (a) an overview of Gallaudet University, focusing on the Social Work Program and the Office of Students with Disabilities program, (b) personal background information about the student and her professor, and (c) perspectives of the educational process by both the student and her instructor. The article concludes with recommendations to both students and instructors for addressing the needs of deaf-blind students in the classroom and university setting. doi:10.1300/J198v06n01_04 *[Article copies available for a fee from The Haworth Document Delivery Service: 1-800-HAWORTH. E-mail address: <docdelivery@ haworthpress.com> Website: <http://www.HaworthPress.com> © 2007 by The Haworth Press, Inc. All rights reserved.]*

Teresa V. Mason, PhD, MSW, is Associate Professor, Department of Social Work, Gallaudet University, 800 Florida Avenue NE, Washington, DC 20002 (E-mail: teresa.mason@gallaudet.edu). Ashleigh Smith, MSW, c/o Gallaudet University, Department of Social Work, 800 Florida Avenue NE, Washington, DC 20002.

[Haworth co-indexing entry note]: "Resources Ancillary Services and Classroom Instruction: Thoughts of a Deaf-Blind Social Work Student and Her Teacher." Mason, Teresa V., and Ashleigh Smith. Co-published simultaneously in *Journal of Social Work in Disability & Rehabilitation* (The Haworth Press, Inc.) Vol. 6, No. 1/2, 2007, pp. 53-65; and: *Disability and Social Work Education: Practice and Policy Issues* (ed: Francis K. O. Yuen, Carol B. Cohen, and Kristine Tower) The Haworth Press, Inc., 2007, pp. 53-65. Single or multiple copies of this article are available for a fee from The Haworth Document Delivery Service [1-800-HAWORTH, 9:00 a.m. - 5:00 p.m. (EST). E-mail address: docdelivery@haworthpress.com].

KEYWORDS. Disability, deaf-blind, resources, services, social work education

INTRODUCTION

In a policy universe that contains people, resources, problems, and solutions, a certain amount of luck is involved in coming up with the right people with the right resources applying the right solutions to the right problems. (Edelman, 2000, pp. 22)

I find that when a student is deaf and blind, the challenges in the classroom for both the student and teacher begin from the minute the class starts, if not before. Imagine my surprise when I arrived to teach my first undergraduate class and saw two deaf-blind students, each with his and her own set of two interpreters. In that moment, I realized that I needed to change my teaching methods. After five years of teaching deaf and deaf-blind students, I find that sometimes a little creativity is involved on the parts of the student and instructor in order to make even a single classroom lecture flow. Sometimes resources are needed to make the system work. At other times, I am convinced, a certain amount of luck and timing is critical.

The purpose of this article is to share my experiences of teaching and a deaf-blind student's experiences of learning in a social work program. This article consists of several parts. First, I provide a basic overview of Gallaudet University, focusing on two programs: the Social Work Program, and the Office of Students With Disabilities (OSWD) program. Second, Ash and I provide information about our personal backgrounds. Third, Ash and I discuss our perspectives of the educational process. Finally, Ash and I offer recommendations to both students and instructors about addressing the needs of deaf-blind students in the classroom and university setting.

GALLAUDET UNIVERSITY SYSTEM

Gallaudet University is a liberal arts college that was founded in 1864 and is located in Washington, DC. In many ways, Gallaudet is similar to other colleges and universities in its function and purpose. However, what makes Gallaudet unique is that it educates deaf and hard of hearing students, making it the only liberal arts college for the deaf in the world (Gallaudet University, 2004).

Communication is an integral part of Gallaudet's mission. Gallaudet recognizes the ". . . right and responsibility to understand and be understood. Clear and well-paced visual communication is a requirement for this learning community. We respect the sign language style of every individual and use whatever is necessary to communicate in a given situation" (Gallaudet, 2004).

OFFICE FOR STUDENTS WITH DISABILITIES (OSWD)

Similar to other universities, Gallaudet offers an ancillary service via the Office for Students With Disabilities (OSWD). While other university student services may provide interpreters and accommodations for deaf students as well as other students with special needs, Gallaudet's support services are specifically for students with low vision and blindness, students with learning disabilities, and students with neurological/orthopedic difficulties (OSWD, 2004). OSWD supports student independence and autonomy ". . . through the provision of reasonable accommodations, academic support groups, self-advocacy, and compensatory training" (OSWD, 2004).

OSWD provides multiple services, including assessment, academic support services, student education and development, professional development and technical assistance, specialized materials and equipment, and special needs information and referral services. In particular, deaf-blind students may utilize note-taking services, interpreting services, orientation and mobility training, Braille and large print services, reader services, low vision equipment and computers, and seeing eye dog programs.

THE SOCIAL WORK PROGRAM

Gallaudet University offers BSW and MSW degrees in its social work program. Ten full-time faculty members teach in the department, five of whom are deaf or hard of hearing. All members of the department use sign language as the primary mode of instruction in the classroom. Because the department is small, a faculty member can easily discuss classroom issues in department or program meetings as well as individually with other colleagues.

For new faculty, the small department offers a chance to brainstorm and solve problems that may arise in the course of teaching. Program meetings and discussions addressed deaf-blind related issues such as classroom accommodations for interpreters, lending textbooks to OSWD for Braille-typing, coordination of deaf-blind interpreters, modification of classroom materials and tests, transportation services to internships, and coordinating interpreters at internship sites. I found these discussions particularly useful because every faculty member in the department had some experience with teaching deaf-blind students. I realized from these discussions that every faculty member had to creatively design an individual education protocol for their particular students. In other words, there was no standard practice of educating deaf-blind students. In the end, I blended the ideas that other colleagues offered in combination with my own to create individual lesson plans to meet the needs of my deaf-blind students.

Background

I met Ashleigh Smith in the fall of 2003 when she became a student in my Research Methods class. Ash was one of two deaf-blind students in my class. Between the two students, they shared a team of three interpreters. That semester I taught a record number of deaf undergraduate students for the class. There were 23 students in the class, 26 individuals including the interpreters.

Immediately I was taken with Ash. She seemed to be a serious student overall. I knew her grade point average was very close to a 4.0. Ash immediately requested a meeting to discuss her learning needs. This young woman, I thought, had been around the block. She was a natural social worker in the making. Allow me to introduce Ash and myself in more detail.

Ashleigh Smith

Ashleigh Smith was almost 24 years old and was a recent BSW graduate from the social work program at Gallaudet University. When she was two and a half years old, she became ill with spinal meningitis. Her illness and a subsequent brain inflammation led to her becoming deaf.

After complaining of sore eyes at the age of six, Ash went to an emergency room where she was given an MRI. Doctors discovered that Ash had a brain tumor that later disappeared inexplicably. However, she began to gradually lose her vision. Initially Ash took steroids, which restored her vision completely. After she experienced another episode of vision loss, the steroids were ineffective. Eventually Ash lost all of the vision in her right eye and some in the left.

At five years old, Ash went to a private Christian school where she learned to lip-read. When her vision began to fail, Ash's parents enrolled her in a homebound schooling program with a teacher who came to her home to teach. Eventually Ash entered the public school system with a sign language interpreter.

In 2001, Ashleigh transferred to Gallaudet University from the Stephen F. Austin State University (SFA). As a result of her experiences as a deaf-blind woman, Ash decided upon a career in social work:

> Throughout the course of my lifetime with the consequences of being deaf-blind, my daily agenda always consisted of challenges with different social systems. I became increasingly frustrated with these systems that I felt were not giving me complete information about what my options were for independent living. I soon discovered that because they wanted to protect me, they sometimes hid information that would have allowed me to do things they did not want me to do.

Teresa Crowe

In 1999, I was hired as an adjunct professor in the Social Work Department at Gallaudet University. I was thrilled because when I began my doctoral program at the University of Maryland in 1997, my eye was on only one prize–a job at Gallaudet. As an alumnus of the MSW program at Gallaudet, my dream was to become a professor there.

I was hired to teach my first class in the Social Work Program in the spring semester in 1999. I was challenged; the learning curve steep. However, the moment I stepped into the classroom to teach the advanced year research course, I knew I had found my place. After 12 years of direct social work practice, 11 of which were in the deaf community, I decided with conviction that I wanted to enter the field of social work education. I sighed in relief to know that my doctoral studies would be put to good use.

That spring semester went by quickly. I practiced the skills I learned from my doctoral class in teaching: how to develop lesson plans and to use PowerPoint. I learned classroom management techniques and developed a fair grading system. I decided to pass out class notes and create interactive activities to help with learning. I told funny stories about my experiences with research. We played research games, like investing their fake $10,000 into the best research proposal presentation. Overall, I strove toward establishing a classroom milieu that was conducive to learning and social interaction. However, in the fall semester of 1999, I realized that the world of social work education was much larger.

In the fall of 1999, I taught a large undergraduate class of approximately 16 students. Students sat in a semi-circle while I stood in front. The reason for this was to allow access to visual communication. All of the students used sign language; so, the beginning of class was always used for moving chairs to ensure that everyone was able to see each other and the teacher. Visual instruction, I had learned from the previous semester, was critical. I handed out notes to the class so that they could watch each other and me without breaking to look down and write notes. When I walked into the classroom that semester, I was in for a big surprise. At opposite ends of the semi-circle sat two deaf-blind students, each with his/her own set of two interpreters. This experience was only the beginning in learning to be flexible, creative, and innovative in classroom teaching.

Now that I described Ash's and my background, let me paint a portrait of the context in which we met. In the following sections, I provide an overview of Gallaudet University. In particular, I focus on two programs in the university that seem most relevant to this chapter: the Office for Students with Disabilities (OSWD) and the Social Work Program.

EDUCATIONAL EXPERIENCES

From our experiences during the 2003-2004 academic year, Ash and I identified three major areas for discussion: resources, ancillary services, and classroom instruction. Each area greatly impacted the learning environment.

RESOURCES

Academic resources and their allocation are issues that every institution must face. Gallaudet University is not different in that regard. The resources of particular interest here are interpreters and computer technology.

Soon after arriving to Gallaudet, Ash became familiar with the Gallaudet Interpreting Services (GIS). Ash reported that the interpreter services were helpful. In particular, she indicated that students were asked which interpreters they preferred and attempted to place these interpreters in her classes. This method of classroom assignment for interpreters empowered students to choose those interpreters with skills that best fit their individual needs.

As the classroom instructor, I found Ash's interpreters indispensable. I introduced myself at the first class meeting and asked them what kinds of materials they needed from me. Sometimes classroom interpreters asked for a copy of the syllabus. Sometimes they asked for a copy of lecture notes or assignments. I made sure all my classroom materials were available for the interpreters. I found that in addition to developing a relationship with Ash, I also needed to develop a sound working relationship with the interpreters.

In addition, I addressed communication and physical space needs with the interpreters and Ash. Typically one interpreter sat next to me in a chair and translated the signs of other students. The other interpreter sat next to Ash and translated my lectures to her. Occasionally when classroom discussion became energized and students' signs overlapped, the interpreters would interrupt to ask for a slow-down of discussion. In this way, Ash was able to understand the conversations.

Ash also needed additional resources for her field placement. Ash needed assistance with transportation not only to the internship site itself, but also to community forums and meetings held outside. Sometimes Ash was unable to attend meetings because there was no interpreter available. Because Ash did not have interpreters with her full-time at the internship site, she was faced with challenges when a hearing person walked into the office to inquire about services.

Another important resource for academic success was computer technology. Initially, Ash discovered immediate challenges with resources.

> I soon discovered that aside from two computers in the library, none of the computers on campus had large print software for the visually impaired. I began to realize that I would have to start again as I had the entrance to every school–junior high, high school, SFA, and now Gallaudet.

Ash was referred to a liaison from the Academic Technology Department who worked with OSWD. After two months of discussion about which administrative department would cover the cost, the software was purchased. In the meantime, Ash used her home computer and software. Clearly, Ash's access to academic resources was severely limited.

Another difficulty with computer technology was software incompatibility. The two computers in the library used a software program called MAGIC, but often did not work well with word processing programs and Internet access. Ash discovered a problem with program incompatibility when she took her required foreign language, Spanish. The department used MAC computers, but the Zoomtext software program, a software program that enlarges text on a computer screen, only ran on IBM compatible computers.

Ash also required Zoomtext at the internship site. One might think that it should be a simple matter of ordering the software and installing it on the agency's computer. I found out quickly that this was more complicated. First, there was discussion between the Academic Technology Department at the university and OSWD about the cost of software. Finally, one of the two departments agreed to pay for the software, but it took several weeks to get to that point. The second hurdle was allowing the software to be installed on government computers (her internship was at the Governor's Office for Deaf and Hard of Hearing located in Baltimore, Maryland). Because of the secure nature of the computer system, special permission was required before installing the software. Meanwhile, Ash was left without computer resources at her agency.

The resource issue at the university was significant because sometimes Ash was unable to complete assignments on time. Conceivably, there was the potential that she may not have been able to complete assignments at all if the resources were not obtained in a timely fashion. When these situations occurred, I waived my late assignment penalty of 10% per missed class to accommodate Ash's needs.

ANCILLARY SERVICES

Ancillary services were critical in meeting Ash's educational needs. In addition to the Gallaudet Interpreting Services, mentioned above, the Office for Students With Disabilities (OSWD) provides multiple services to students with disabilities. It is unreasonable to think that small ancillary departments can address every accommodation necessary for students, and do it in record time. Again, in a perfect world, we, as instructors, would like to have the resources and services in place prior to the first class meeting. Some accommodations can be arranged prior to that first class. For example, Ash arranged for her classroom interpreters so when the first day of class arrived, so did she along with two personal interpreters. Other ancillary services were not so easy. Ash reported feeling frustrated by this.

> [OSWD] asked for the [text] books from professors and then began typing each word into a word processor. At SFA [Stephen F. Austin State University], books were utilized and then were copied on a copier to make large print books held together by ring or spiral bindings. This procedure allowed them to have the books ready at the beginning of each semester. As for OSWD, I always had to drop in to ask if the next chapter was ready or not during the course of a semester. This was not ideal for me as I do my studying at my own time and if the chapters were not ready for me, then that put me in a position where time did not serve me. After the first semester, I decided that I would rely heavily on my closed circuit television (CCTV) instead of OSWD to better manage my time.

Usually over the semester break, be it winter or summer, OSWD asks to borrow my class textbooks so they can begin typing. This is a tricky question because if I lend out my only copies of the texts, then I don't have the resources I need to develop the lectures for class. This system of "robbing Peter to pay Paul" created stress for both Ash and me. Ash often expressed frustration to me about not having the chapters and articles she needed in order to complete the homework, quizzes, tests, and projects. Again, flexibility on my part to allow Ash to complete assignments, tests, and readings at a different pace was needed.

Another service provided by OSWD is note taking. Ash stated that note-taking services were often delayed and did not begin until after the semester started. She reported up to two months of waiting before notetakers were hired. By that time, Ash noted, note-taking services were useless.

Ash reported that at her former university, SFA, note-takers were provided with laptops. Ash enjoyed this service because she was not faced with the problem of trying to decipher illegible writing. Notes were saved onto floppy disks and given to Ash at the end of class. She compared her experience at SFA with Gallaudet, where note-takers were not permitted to use the university's laptops. Ash found herself unable to read the note-takers' writing and asked her classmates for assistance.

OSWD also provided Ash with transportation and training to attend her field internship site. Ash reported that the Orientation and Mobility

(O & M) services provided by OSWD were helpful with internship placement.

> Without O & M, I would not have been able to succeed in traveling to and from the Office of Deaf and Hard of Hearing.

There were instances when Ash was unable to attend her internship because of inclement weather. Sometimes there were community forums and meetings that Ash was unable to attend because of difficulty with transportation. Ash often balanced her work needs with the availability of a train schedule or cab fare in order to meet her internship duties. Flexibility in scheduling and attending meetings was necessary.

Overall, the ancillary services from OSWD provide necessary and important services to support students' needs. Ash received a great deal of support from OSWD. Ash and I identified areas of improvement for the services, but were thankful for the help that was provided.

CLASSROOM INSTRUCTION

As any student and teacher know, the classroom is where the action starts. Students become active and interactive learners in the classroom. Teachers utilize skill and technique to convey their knowledge to the students. There are special concerns, though, when deaf-blind students are involved.

Ash identified two major concerns with classroom instruction: communication and independent mobility. For communication, Ash expressed continued frustration about her classmates' forgetfulness about having a deaf-blind student in class. She reported that at times students would engage in energetic communication with several students signing simultaneously. The classroom interpreters were unable to capture the conversations completely, thereby leaving Ash without the full benefit of discussion.

As her instructor, I took responsibility for controlling the classroom discussion. Sometimes I was more successful than at other times. Sometimes the interpreters interrupted the conversation so they could catch up for Ash's understanding. I always tried to support the interpreters in this. Often I found myself engaged with the class at large, not paying attention to the pace and flow of the interpreters. However, when the interpreters interrupted, I recognized this as if Ash herself had raised her hand for clarification. I found that balancing students needs as a general issue required skill and creativity in teaching. I tried to be fully aware that there were special circumstances in the class and reminded students frequently as well.

My students often report that my research classes are challenging given the best of circumstances. I ask them to become actively involved in the research process so they can get a better grasp of the esoteric concepts we discuss. Collecting observational data is one of the easier assignments in class, one which students seem to enjoy. However, how can a deaf-blind student collect observational data? The deaf students collect data on campus, but then again, all the students sign on campus. So, they can be observed. Deaf-blind students cannot observe conversations as the other students can. As an alternative, I asked the student about having the interpreters simply translate what's happening in the environment. The deaf-blind student, along with the other students, is still expected to write field notes and attempt to analyze the data collected. The task is a formidable one, especially for deaf-blind students.

Course content was also an issue that needed my attention. While I could not adapt the content for a particular student, I tried to teach it in "user-friendly ways." Ash noted in particular that the research classes were challenging for her as a deaf-blind student.

> For Crowe's first data research course, my primary concern was the observations she assigned us to perform. Since observations rely on the use of vision, I was not sure how best to go about doing them. I remember asking [another deaf-blind student] what he would propose and he mentioned to me what Crowe had suggested to him–that his interpreters could tell him what they were seeing in his environment. I used that to do the observations and while this was helpful–I wondered if this was the realistic way to do actual and formal observations.

Ash said the data analysis course with its statistical content was especially difficult. She reported that the course content was paced fast and that she had difficulty keeping up. Ash reported that she did not benefit from the weekly Supplemental Instruction sessions (a lab designed to reinforce learning) because she found the group format difficult.

I found other ways to modify my teaching approaches for Ash. She identified two aspects of her classroom learning that she found helpful: instructors' use of PowerPoint and small class size. While I was unable to control the size of her particular class, I used PowerPoint for classroom instruction. I gave her copies of the lectures as well as copies of my teaching notes. Classmates also provided Ash with PowerPoint copies from their presentations and projects.

However, there were moments in the lectures, especially when I saw that students were having a hard time grasping a concept, when I ad-libbed. I created new data, like the number of times college students kiss when first dating. These types of ad-libs served first as an attention grabber, then were used to apply methodological discussions. This type of impromptu lecturing often made a boring lull in the classroom exciting and energized the class. However, it put additional strain on Ash because she did not have the visual information prior to class.

Classroom interaction is vital to the learning process. Ash and I both worked to be as prepared as possible for the learning activities and discussions. Even with the best intentions, issues arose in the classroom that was unforeseen. Advance preparation and attention to detail help to create an environment for a deaf-blind student that is conducive to learning.

CONCLUSION

Ash and I both recognize that there are difficult situations in social work education that require flexibility, patience, and creativity on both the parts of the teacher and of the student. Ash and I agree that there are systematic and financial constraints on creating true, satisfying accessibility to education. We see that there are true limits to financial availability. There is limited knowledge of the players in the academic environment. There are moments of individual oversight and inadequate preparation. The situation is not dire, though. There are many solutions that can remedy particular problems in the classroom and learning experience. Here are some of our recommendations:

- Allow deaf-blind students and instructors to creatively construct learning experiences that address the learning objectives. Understand that the ways the learning objectives are achieved for deaf-blind students may not be identical to the other students'.
- When possible, be sensitive to class size when deaf-blind students are in the group. The larger the group, the more difficult it is for deaf-blind students to participate.
- Remind other students repeatedly, if necessary, that communication must be structured and orderly in order to accommodate the deaf-blind student.
- Become familiar with the academic ancillary services.

- When possible, instructors prepare learning materials in advance and give to the deaf-blind students.
- When possible, deaf-blind students meet with the instructors before classes start. Provide the instructors with written guidelines about how they can make the learning experience better.

Above all, I think that it is important for instructors and students alike to communicate openly and honestly. I encourage students to discuss the learning objectives and how they are achieved. I encourage instructors to seek support when challenges appear overwhelming. I have found that sometimes there are helpers in disguise. At other times there can be just plain luck.

REFERENCES

Edelman, I. (2000). Evaluation and community-based initiatives. *Social Policy, 31*(2), 13-23.

Gallaudet University. (2004). Homepage. Retrieved June 29, 2004, from http://www. gallaudet.edu/thegallaudetexperience.htm

Office for Students with Disabilities (2003). Services and Assistances. Retrieved June 29, 2004, from http://depts.gallaudet.edu/oswd/services.htm

Office for Students with Disabilities (2004). About the OSWD. Retrieved June 29, 2004, from http://depts.gallaudet.edu/oswd/about.htm

doi:10.1300/J198v06n01_04

An Overview of and Comments on the Americans With Disabilities Act (ADA)

John T. Pardeck

Jean A. Pardeck

SUMMARY. The authors overview the key components of the ADA in this article. A discussion is offered on why and how persons with disabilities are discriminated against. Critical United States Supreme Court decisions are presented; these decisions have greatly limited the power of the ADA in protecting the rights of persons with disabilities. Even though the United States Supreme Court has narrowed the impact of the ADA in American life, a number of Equal Employment Opportunity Commission (EEOC) cases are presented suggesting this federal agency is attempting to protect persons with disabilities against discrimination. Finally, the authors deal with the topic of advocacy; advocacy may well be one of the most effective tools to help insure that the rights of people with disabilities are protected. doi:10.1300/J198v06n01_05 *[Article copies available for a fee from The Haworth Document Delivery Service: 1-800-HAWORTH. E-mail address: <docdelivery@haworthpress.com> Website: <http://www.HaworthPress.com> © 2007 by The Haworth Press, Inc. All rights reserved.]*

John T. Pardeck, PhD, MSW (1947-2004), was Emeritus Professor, Department of Social Work, Missouri State University, and Jean A. Pardeck, MEd, is Reading Specialist, 2022 East Barataria, Springfield, MO 65804 (E-mail: pardecks@hotmail.com).

[Haworth co-indexing entry note]: "An Overview of and Comments on the Americans With Disabilities Act (ADA)." Pardeck, John T., and Jean A. Pardeck. Co-published simultaneously in *Journal of Social Work in Disability & Rehabilitation* (The Haworth Press, Inc.) Vol. 6, No. 1/2, 2007, pp. 67-91; and: *Disability and Social Work Education: Practice and Policy Issues* (ed: Francis K. O. Yuen, Carol B. Cohen, and Kristine Tower) The Haworth Press, Inc., 2007, pp. 67-91. Single or multiple copies of this article are available for a fee from The Haworth Document Delivery Service [1-800-HAWORTH, 9:00 a.m. - 5:00 p.m. (EST). E-mail address: docdelivery@haworthpress.com].

KEYWORDS. ADA, persons with disabilities, US Supreme Court, EEOC, advocacy

INTRODUCTION

On July 26, 1990, the Americans With Disabilities Act (ADA) was signed into law by President George H. Bush. Referred to as the "emancipation proclamation for the disabled," this legislation is of great importance to the 43 million members of American society with disabling conditions. The ADA has significant implications for all citizens, not only those with disabilities. The ADA also has significance for how social work agencies and other systems operate (Pardeck, 1998). For example, local governments have been required to make changes in countless ordinances, building codes and policies. These changes must also be made by public social work agencies. Many changes have been required of private industry, including the for-profit social work agencies, to be in compliance with the ADA. These include hiring procedures, job restructuring, work schedules, training materials and equipment used, and other factors affecting persons with disabilities working in or coming in contact with the private sector (Pardeck, 1998). The ADA, therefore, has profound implications for all aspects of American life including the profession of social work.

BACKGROUND ON THE AMERICANS
WITH DISABILITIES ACT

The ADA is grounded in a philosophy that views unequal treatment of persons with disabilities as a violation of their human rights. The ADA is based on the position that persons with disabilities have not received the same treatment as others, and that it is the responsibility of the state to affirm or re-affirm those rights through judicial and legislative actions (Pardeck, 1998). People with disabilities are viewed as having intrinsic worth and dignity. Yet a utilitarian theme also guides the ADA, with employers being required to make reasonable accommodations to assist the person with a disability in the workplace. The cost for accommodating the person with a disability cannot necessarily outweigh the benefits. This utilitarian view always stresses the practicality and cost effectiveness of programs (Pardeck, 1998).

Findings Supporting Need for the ADA

The ADA (P.L. Law 101-336, 1990) was signed into law based on the following findings:

1. There are 43 million Americans who have one or more physical or mental disabilities.
2. Historically society has tended to isolate and segregate the disabled.
3. Discrimination in the areas of employment, housing, public accommodations, transportation, and education has been an incredible deterrent in the implementation of the rights of the disabled.
4. Discrimination on the basis of disability frequently had no legal recourse.
5. Individuals with disabilities are intentionally excluded by architectural, transportation or communication barriers, and practices that result in lesser opportunities.
6. People with disabilities as a group occupy inferior status and are disadvantaged socially, vocationally, economically, and educationally.
7. Individuals with disabilities are a distinct and insular minority who have been faced with restrictions and limitations and subjected to unequal treatment.
8. The nation's proper goals should be to assure equality of opportunity, full participation, independent living, and economic self-sufficiency.
9. The continued existence of unfair and unnecessary discrimination against the disabled denies them the opportunity to compete, and costs the United States billions of dollars in unnecessary expenses resulting from dependency and nonproductivity (Pardeck, 1998).

Purposes of the ADA

There are four purposes of the ADA based upon the nine findings:

1. To provide a national mandate to eliminate discrimination against individuals with disabilities.
2. To provide an enforceable standard addressing discrimination.
3. To ensure that the federal government will play a central role in enforcing these standards.
4. To involve congressional authority in order to address the major areas of discrimination faced by people with disabilities (Pardeck, 1998).

Defining Disability

For an individual to be defined as disabled under the ADA, he or she must meet one or more of the following descriptions (The Americans With Disabilities Act P.L. Law 101-336, 1990, p. 6):

1. Has a physical or mental impairment that substantially limits one or more of the major life activities, or
2. Has a record of such an impairment, or
3. Is regarded as having such an impairment.

Major life activities include but are not limited to walking, speaking, seeing, hearing, breathing, learning, working, reproduction and caring for oneself (Pardeck, 1998).

The ADA does not offer a specific list of disabilities that it covers. The reason for not offering a list is noted in a 1989 report (The Americans With Disabilities Act of 1989, p. 22) from the United States Senate:

> It is not possible to include in the (ADA) legislation a list of all the specific conditions, diseases, or infections that would constitute physical or mental impairments because of the difficulty of ensuring the comprehensiveness of such a list, particularly in light of the fact that new disorders may develop in the future. The term includes, however, such conditions, diseases and infections as orthopedic, visual, speech, and hearing impairment, cerebral palsy, epilepsy, muscular dystrophy, multiple sclerosis, infections with the human immunodeficiency virus (HIV), cancer, heart disease, diabetes, mental retardation, emotional illness, and specific learning disabilities.

It is an extremely complex process to define a disability under the ADA. Furthermore, traditional stereotypes for disabilities have been challenged by the definition of disability under the ADA; many professionals including social workers view a disability as simply a visible physical impairment (Pardeck, 1998). However, a disability is also defined under the ADA as a person with a record of an impairment or being regarded as having an impairment. The second and third prongs of the definition of a disability involve extremely complex legal issues that call for training and education of professionals working with people with disabilities. Research concludes that a record of a disability or being regarded as having a disability can result in discrimination.

Prior to the 1990s, an employer could simply fire an employee because the person was a cancer survivor. Such behavior is now a violation of the ADA. Cancer survivors, like many other persons with disabilities, are five times more likely to be fired or laid off than other employees (Arnold, 1999). Research also shows that up to 50 percent of cancer survivors feel they are discriminated against in the workplace because they had cancer (Arnold, 1999).

Examples of why cancer survivors are confronted with job discrimination include the following beliefs and stereotypes (Pardeck, 1998):

1. Cancer survivors are viewed as having higher rates of absenteeism than other employees; this is not supported by fact.
2. Many employers have a traditional view of cancer; they think cancer means death, not realizing that many cancers can be cured or controlled.
3. Some employers discriminate against cancer survivors because they do not feel comfortable having them in the workplace. This is a common problem for people confronted with other kinds of disabilities as well.
4. Some employers feel that cancer survivors will drive their health care costs up; again this is not based on fact.

The above beliefs about cancer survivors are very similar to the stereotypes often used to justify discrimination against other groups of persons with disabilities. The ADA is an important federal law that is helping to change these stereotypes (Pardeck, 2002b).

Major Titles of the ADA

There are five major titles under the Americans With Disabilities Act. These are:

Title I. Discrimination Regarding Employment. This Title defines and describes how employers are prohibited from discriminating against a qualified individual with a disability in all terms and conditions of employment. This Title has the greatest importance for employee selection.

Title II. Public Services. This Title prohibits discrimination and increases the accessibility of persons with disabilities to programs run by state and local governments. For the field of social work this includes public social work agencies, colleges and universities. This title also requires that public transportation become accessible to people with disabilities.

Title III. Private Accommodations and Services. This Title requires that private businesses serving the public make their goods and services available to people with disabilities.

Title IV. The Telecommunications Title. This Title requires that telephone services be accessible to people with hearing and speech impairments by providing them with relay services. The relay service uses an operator as an intermediary communicator between the hearing person and the individual needing assistance.

Title V. Miscellaneous. This Title prohibits retaliation against an individual because of actions related to the Act, and provides information on the implementation of the ADA, the Rehabilitation Act of 1973, and state laws (Pardeck, 1998).

Title I (Employment)

The first significant national legislation to protect people with disabilities was the Rehabilitation Act of 1973. This act, however, only covers those entities that receive federal contracts or subcontracts exceeding a certain dollar amount. Serving as the model for the Americans With Disabilities Act, including Title I of the ADA, the Rehabilitation Act provided the definition for a disability under the ADA.

Title I of the ADA covers all employers, both public and private, who employ 15 or more workers (Pardeck, 1998). Long a problem for people with disabilities, the goal of Title I is to prevent employment discrimination.

Discrimination against people with disabilities in the workplace occurs in many different forms. The discrimination is sometimes intentional, sometimes unintentional. Much of the discrimination against people with disabilities is a result of able people seeing the disabled as different from others. As children, most people often experienced educational systems that segregated people with disabilities from others. This kind of segregation also extended into the workplace, for example, the placement of persons with disabilities in Sheltered Workshops (Pardeck, 1998). Our lack of awareness of people with disabilities and their special needs has been increased by this kind of segregation. The differences of people with disabilities and the able are emphasized and not their similarities. Segregation of people with disabilities in schools and the workplace has increased able persons' fears and discomfort with people who have disabilities (Pardeck, 1998).

Aimed at changing the historical patterns of excluding people with disabilities from the workplace, the objective of Title I is to place people with disabilities into meaningful employment and to offer them better job opportunities. Once people with disabilities have achieved greater integration into the workplace, many of the misconceptions about people with disabilities will be eliminated (Pardeck, 1998).

To comply with Title I, employers must make sure that the employee selection process and the requirements of the ADA in the area of employment are clearly understood by all employees. The employment provisions of the ADA cover hiring, promotions, pay, firing, job training, benefits, and virtually all aspects of the workplace. National legislators recognized that they could not predict every possible form of employment discrimination, so they created a law that is broad and open to interpretation. An important component of Title I is defining who is protected and outlining the basic responsibilities of employers (Pardeck, 1998).

Employers must also understand that Title I includes a definition for not only a disability under the law, but also for what is meant by a qualified individual with a disability. A qualified individual with a disability under the employment provisions of the ADA is as follows (Equal Employment Opportunity Commission & U. S. Department of Justice, 1992):

> A qualified individual with a disability is a person who meets legitimate skill, experience, education, or other requirements of an employment position that s/he holds or seeks, and who can perform the "essential" functions of the position with or without reasonable accommodation. Requiring the ability to perform "essential" functions assures that an individual with a disability will not be considered unqualified simply because of inability to perform marginal or incidental job functions. (p. 2)

If an individual is qualified to perform essential job functions except for limitations caused by a disability, the employer must consider whether the individual could perform these functions with a reasonable accommodation. A written job description that has been prepared in advance of advertising or interviewing applicants for a job will be considered as evidence, although not conclusive evidence, of the essential functions of the job (Pardeck, 1998).

Essential functions of a job include the fundamental duties required of a position. These qualifications include educational requirements, work experience, training levels, job skills, licensing and certification requirements, and other job related requirements determined by the employer (Pardeck, 1998).

The ADA does not mandate it, but employers should have a complete job description for all positions in an organization including those that

the employer wishes to fill. Employers should list in writing any key duties for a position; these should become a part of the job description. Title I does not require employers to eliminate or make changes to core job
duties or essential functions of the job for the person with a disability
(Pardeck, 1998). Every position, however, typically has several tasks
that are not vital to the position; these tasks are viewed as nonessential
functions. Under the ADA, an employer cannot refuse to hire a person
with a disability because of their inability to do a nonessential task
(Pardeck, 1998).

It is emphasized by Title I that an organization has every right to hire
the most qualified individual. The most qualified individual is obviously
the one who can best perform the essential functions of the job, with or
without accommodations. It is the employer's responsibility to determine
these essential functions. Employers should be prepared, however, to
provide reasonable accommodations to help the person with a disability
perform a job (Pardeck, 1998).

It is critical for the employer to apply hiring criteria consistently to all
applicants, including the able and persons with disabilities, when considering individuals for a position. Qualifications of a job may include
but are not limited to educational requirements, work experience, training skills, and licensing and certification requirements. If a person with
a disability is the most qualified person for a position, that person should
be offered the position. This is equally true for the able person (Pardeck,
1998).

A reasonable accommodation is an important aspect of Title I as well
as other Titles under the ADA. It is a modification or adjustment for a
position, which helps a qualified individual with a disability perform
the tasks of a job. The employer can accommodate both the essential
functions and the nonessential functions of a position (Pardeck, 1998).

Title II (Public Services)

This Title of the ADA prohibits discrimination against persons with
disabilities in all services, programs, and activities provided or made
available by state or local government. In employment, state and local
governments cannot discriminate against job applicants and employees
with disabilities regardless of the number of people they employ (Pardeck,
1998). State and local governments were prohibited from discriminating against persons with disabilities prior to the ADA under Section 504
of the Rehabilitation Act of 1973. Section 504 prohibits discrimination

on the basis of disability in any programs and activities that receive a set amount of federal funds (Pardeck, 1998).

Title II of the ADA, however, extends the nondiscrimination requirements of Section 504 to the activities of all state and local governments, regardless of whether they receive any federal support. Title II has two subtitles, A and B. Subtitle A covers all activities of state and local governments other than public transit. Subtitle B deals with the provision of publicly funded transit (Pardeck, 1998).

Title III (Private Accommodations and Services)

Private accommodations and services are covered by Title III of the ADA. It requires that private businesses serving the public make their goods and services available to people with disabilities. Titles II and III are very similar in scope; however Title II covers state and local governments, where Title III covers private entities (Pardeck, 1998).

Titles IV and V

Title IV of the ADA requires that people with hearing and speech impairments have accessible telephone services by providing them with relay services.

Title V prohibits retaliation against an individual because of actions related to the Act; it also provides information on the implementation of the ADA, the Rehabilitation Act of 1973, and state laws.

DISCRIMINATION ON THE BASIS OF DISABILITY

Harrison and Gilbert (1992) report findings from testimonies made by individuals and representatives of various organizations concerning the need for the passage of the ADA. For example, Timothy Cook of the National Disability Action Center testified (Harrison and Gilbert, 1992):

> As Rosa Parks taught us, and as the Supreme Court ruled thirty-five years ago in Brown vs. Board of Education, segregation "affects one's heart and mind in ways that may never be undone. Separate but equal is inherently unequal." (p. 10)

Others testified that discrimination also included exclusion, or denial of benefits, services, or other opportunities that are as effective and meaningful as those provided to others. Furthermore, discrimination results from actions or inactions that discriminate by effect as well as by intention. Under these circumstances, discrimination includes the lack of access to buildings, standards and criteria, and practices based on thoughtlessness or indifference, that discriminate against persons with disabilities. A number of individuals testified that they were denied jobs because they had AIDS, were former cancer victims, had epilepsy, and other serious illnesses (Harrison and Gilbert, 1992).

People with disabilities are uniquely underprivileged and disadvantaged, according to major public opinion polls such as the Harris poll. They are much poorer, much less educated and have less social life and lower levels of self-satisfaction than other Americans (Harrison and Gilbert, 1992).

All of the data and testimony gathered by the Congress that resulted in the passage of the ADA found that persons with disabilities experience discrimination in virtually every aspect of American life. Individuals with disabilities experience staggering levels of unemployment and poverty. Two-thirds of all people with disabilities between the ages of 16 and 64 are not working at all, yet a large majority of those not working want to work. Sixty-six percent of working-aged people with disabilities who are not working wanted a job. What emerged from the research conducted by Congress was that persons with disabilities were one of the most oppressed minority groups in the United States (Harrison and Gilbert, 1992).

SIGNIFICANT COURT RULINGS AND THE ADA

HIV Infection

Bragdon vs. Abbott (524 U.S. 624, June 25, 1998) resulted in an important ruling by the United States Supreme Court concerning persons who have HIV infection. The Court ruled that a person with HIV infection, even though it has not yet progressed to the so-called symptomatic phase, is disabled under the ADA. The Court also affirmed that patients infected with HIV posed no direct threat to the health and safety of dentists. One could generalize this ruling to health care providers in general (Pardeck, 2002a).

Corrections

In the *Pennsylvania Department of Corrections vs. Yeskey* (524 U.S. 206, June 15, 1998), the United States Supreme Court held that state prison systems must provide reasonable accommodations to prisoners under the ADA. Ronald R. Yeskey was an inmate sentenced to serve 18 to 36 months in a Pennsylvania correctional facility. Mr. Yeskey alleged that exclusion from a Boot Camp because of his hypertension, which would have shortened his sentence, violated the ADA (Pardeck, 2001).

A lower court ruled that Mr. Yeskey was discriminated against under the ADA and that the Pennsylvania Correctional System violated Title II of the ADA which covers state run programs, services, and activities including prisons. The United States Supreme Court upheld the lower court's decision in 1998 (Pardeck, 2001).

Social Security Benefits (SSDI) and the ADA

In *Cleveland vs. Policy Management* (526 U.S. 795, May 24, 1999), the United States Supreme Court reversed a lower federal court decision that held an applicant filing for or receiving SSDI does not automatically bar an individual from filing an ADA lawsuit. The plaintiff in this case, Carolyn Cleveland, experienced a stroke and filed an application for SSDI, in which she indicated that she was disabled and not able to work (Pardeck, 2001).

After filing for SSDI, her condition improved and she returned to work, thus her benefits application was denied. Three months after returning to work, however, she was fired by her employer because she "could no longer do her job because of her condition." After termination, Cleveland asked the Social Security Administration to reconsider her SSDI application (Pardeck, 2002a).

A week before receiving her SSDI benefit award, however, Cleveland filed an ADA lawsuit contending that her employer terminated her without reasonably accommodating her disability by offering additional training and time to complete her work. A federal court ruled in favor of her employer. The lower court concluded that an application for or the receipt of SSDI benefits creates a rebuttable presumption that the claimant is not a qualified person with a disability under the ADA (Pardeck, 2002a).

Cleveland's case was appealed to the United States Supreme Court. Addressing the similarities and differences between the Social Security Act and the ADA, the Supreme Court observed that both laws help individuals with disabilities in different ways. The Social Security Act provides monetary benefits to people who have a disability, while the ADA seeks to eliminate unwarranted discrimination against persons with disabilities. In other words, just because a person applies for or receives SSDI benefits does not automatically mean he or she loses ADA rights (Pardeck, 2001).

Defining a Disability Under the ADA

The United States Supreme Court has attempted to clarify the definition of a disability under the ADA with three rulings that include *Sutton vs. United Air Lines* (527 U.S. 471, June 22, 1999), *Murphy vs. United Parcel Service Incorporated* (527 U.S. 516, June 22, 1998), and *Albertsons Incorporated vs. Kirkingburg* (527 U.S. 555, June 22, 1999).

In *Sutton vs. United Air Lines* (1999), twin sisters on the basis of poor eyesight were denied pilot positions. They had 20/20 corrected vision and had considerable experience as commercial pilots with regional airlines. United Airlines requires pilots to have at least 20/100 vision in each eye without any corrective measures. The sisters claimed that they were covered under the ADA, since without corrective measures their eyesight was weak enough to substantially limit a major life activity, seeing. The airline countered that because their sight was normal with corrective measures, they did not have a disability under the ADA. A lower federal court ruled in favor of United Airlines; the Supreme Court upheld this lower court decision (Pardeck, 2002a).

Murphy vs. United Parcel Service Incorporated (1998) involved Vaughn Murphy, who worked as a mechanic with United Parcel Service. As a mechanic, Murphy was required to have a Department of Transportation (DOT) health card because he needed to drive large trucks for road checks. Murphy's initial physical exam cleared him to work and he was granted a DOT health card and commercial driver's license. A month later, a blood pressure reading showed his blood pressure to be above DOT guidelines; his employer fired him because of this. Murphy claimed he had a disability under the ADA because without medication he would be unable to do major life activities. He argued that United Parcel should allow him to adjust his medication in order to lower his blood pressure to a level acceptable to the DOT health guidelines as a reasonable accommodation. A lower court ruled in favor of the employer, United Parcel. The court held that Murphy was terminated because his blood pressure exceeded the DOT's requirement and therefore he was not a qualified person with a disability. The Supreme Court upheld the lower federal court's ruling (Pardeck, 2002a).

The final employment case involved *Albertsons Incorporated vs. Kirkingburg* (1998). Kirkingburg, a truck driver, passed the necessary

tests for a license despite impaired vision in one eye and was errone-
ously certified by the Department of Transportation and given his commercial truck driver's license. When Kirkingburg was correctly assessed in
1992, he was told that he had to get a waiver from the DOT. Albertsons,
however, fired him for failing to meet the DOT vision standards and refused to rehire him after receiving a waiver.

Kirkingburg filed a job discrimination lawsuit under the ADA against
Albertsons. A lower federal court ruled that Kirkingburg was not a qualified person with a disability. An appeals court ruled that Kirkingburg
had established that he was a person with a disability under the ADA by
demonstrating that the manner in which he sees differed significantly
from the regulations in setting a job-related vision standard. The case
was appealed to the United States Supreme Court, which reversed the
Appeals Court ruling. The Supreme Court held that an employer's right
to set safety guidelines or adhere to federal guidelines was seen as enough
reason to refuse to hire or fire an individual. Furthermore, even if the
DOT waived the sight guidelines on an experimental basis, employers
do not have to waive their safety standards (Pardeck, 2002a).

In *Sutton vs. United Airlines, Murphy vs. United Parcel Service*, and
Alberstons vs. Kirkingburg, the United States Supreme Court ruled
against the plaintiffs in all three employment cases. In the Sutton case,
the Supreme Court found that whether an individual has a disability as
defined by the ADA depends upon the effect of one's condition or impairment "in reference to the measures that mitigate the individual's impairment." This means that individuals should be evaluated on the basis
of their condition with the use of medication or assistive devices when
determining whether their disability substantially limits major life functioning. The United States Supreme Court used the same line of reason-
ing in *Murphy vs. United Parcel Service* and *Alberstons vs. Kirkingburg*
(Pardeck, 2001).

Board of Trustees vs. Garrett

In the *Board of Trustees of the University of Alabama vs. Garrett*
(531 U.S. 356, Feb 21, 2001), the question answered was whether the
11th Amendment bars employees of a state from recovering monetary
damages from the state for violations of Title I of the ADA. The Court
held that suits by state employees to recover money damages from the
state for violations of Title I of the ADA are barred by the 11th Amendment. However, in footnote 9 of the opinion, the Court indicated that Title I of the ADA is still applicable to the states, and can be enforced by

the United States in actions for money damages. Regardless of this foot-note in the opinion, the Court greatly weakened the protections of state employees under Title I of the ADA (Pardeck, 2002a).

Olmstead vs. L.C.

Olmstead vs. L.C. (527 U.S. 581, June 22, 1998) has implications for persons with disabilities receiving services from state and local govern-ment. The plaintiffs in this case were two intellectually and emotionally impaired patients who were institutionalized in the state of Georgia. They claimed that they were denied services in the most integrated set-ting because they were placed in a state operated institution and were thus segregated from the rest of society. The doctors for the plaintiffs found that community based services were more appropriate for their treatment needs (Pardeck, 2002a).

A lower federal court ruled in favor of the plaintiffs, finding that a core principle underlying the ADA was violated, that being to integrate persons with disabilities into the larger society. *Olmstead vs. L. C.* was appealed to the Supreme Court; the Court ruled that the institutiona-lization of mentally disabled people is a form of discrimination and that the state of Georgia violated the plaintiff's rights under the ADA (Pardeck, 2001).

The rulings by the United States Supreme Court over the last 10 years have had a profound impact on the ADA. Even though a number of these rulings have strengthened some aspects of the ADA, others have greatly limited the impact of the ADA. Specifically, the definition of a disabil-ity has been narrowed. Title I now only provides limited protection for state employees. In *Tennessee vs. Lane*, currently before the Court, a ruling in favor of the State of Tennessee will mean states will no longer have to insure that government buildings and programs need to be ac-cessible to persons with disabilities. These recent court rulings have im-portant implications for social workers and other professionals working in social services (Pardeck, 2002a).

THE EQUAL EMPLOYMENT OPPORTUNITY COMMISSON (EEOC) ENFORCEMENT OF TITLE I

Since the passage of the ADA, the EEOC has taken an active and forceful role in removing barriers and increasing opportunities for peo-ple with disabilities in the workplace. Nearly a quarter of the EEOC's caseload is comprised of discrimination complaints under Title I of the ADA. The EEOC has taken a number of ADA employment cases to court; the agency prevailed in nearly 90 percent of these cases. There have been 126,000 charges of discrimination under Title I; 15 percent have been resolved in favor of the individual. Since the enactment of the ADA, $261 million in payments and other benefits have been won by the EEOC for persons with disabilities in the workplace. Keep in mind that prior to the enactment of the ADA, a person with a disability could be terminated from a job because of a disability. Such behavior by an employer is now illegal under the ADA (Castro, 2000).

Many individuals with disabilities have received monetary and non-monetary benefits through the enforcement efforts of the EEOC. The following are examples of some of the cases that were settled by the EEOC without using litigation (Castro, 2000):

- A large drug store chain changed its job application form by removing unlawful pre-employment inquiries about applicants' disabilities.
- A defense contractor agreed to change its policy requiring employees to disclose their use of prescription medication on an ongoing basis.
- A state law requiring a GED or high school diploma for day care positions was changed to recognize "Certificate of Learning" granted to individuals with intellectual disabilities.
- For a person with diabetes, who was denied a position as a firefighter, his medical condition was found to pose no threat: he was hired and provided monetary relief.
- A person with disfigurement of her face and head, denied a job at a bookstore though qualified, was given the job and provided monetary relief.

The EEOC has filed 416 lawsuits on behalf of persons with disabilities. The following summarizes some of these important lawsuits (Castro, 2000):

- The very first lawsuit filed by the EEOC under the ADA was the EEOC and *Charles Wessel vs. AIC Security Investigation, Ltd.* Charles Wessel, fired from his position because he had terminal brain cancer, was awarded $22,000 in back pay, $50,000 in compensatory damages, and $150,000 in punitive damages.

- The Commission in *EEOC vs. Professional Nurses, Inc.* won a verdict in favor of a highly qualified nurse who was denied employment because of her history of schizophrenia.
- In the *EEOC vs. Union Carbide*, the Commission sued Union Carbide when it refused to provide a reasonable accommodation for an employee with a bipolar disorder. The employee had requested that he be assigned to a non-rotating shift schedule; he was awarded $120,000 in compensatory damages and Union Carbide agreed to provide accommodations for employees with disabilities in the future.
- A jury found that a custodian with mental retardation was fired because of his disability in *EEOC vs. Showbiz Pizza Time, Inc.* A manager stated he did not want his company to employ "those type of people." The fired employee was awarded $70,000 in compensatory damages for emotional distress and 13 million in punitive damages, which was later reduced, as well as back pay and the reinstatement of the employee.
- In *EEOC vs. The Kroger Company*, a favorable verdict resulted for a cashier with paraplegia who could not use the store's restroom or breakroom because they were located down a flight of stairs. The company agreed to build an accessible bathroom and breakroom and also provided the employee with $225,000 in compensatory and punitive damages.
- In *EEOC vs. El Chico Restaurants of Louisiana, Inc.*, the Commission challenged a restaurant's refusal to hire a job applicant as a dishwasher because he was blind. During the job interview the applicant was not even allowed to demonstrate how he could do the job. The restaurant agreed to provide the applicant with $24,000 in monetary relief and to provide training for all its managers on issues related to the ADA.
- The Commission claimed in *EEOC vs. Guardmark* that a security guard was fired because he had insulin-dependent diabetes. The company reimbursed the guard $25,000 in back pay and compensatory damages and donated $25,000 to a scholarship fund for persons with disabilities.
- In *EEOC vs. Armstrong Brothers Tool Company*, the Commission challenged the company's firing of a sales representative because he had epilepsy and previously had surgery for a brain tumor. The company agreed to pay the former employee $27,000 in back pay and $108,000 in compensatory damages.

ADVOCACY AND THE AMERICANS
WITH DISABILITIES ACT

The Americans With Disabilities Act, like other civil rights legislation of the past, is aimed at an oppressed group, persons with disabilities, who have been denied equal opportunity to participate in American society (Pardeck, 1998).

Like other oppressed groups within American society, people with disabilities have suffered tremendous discrimination (Ianacone, 1977). The National Council on Disability, the Civil Rights Commission, and national polls all conclude that discrimination against people with disabilities is pervasive in American society (Pardeck & Chung, 1992). This discrimination is sometimes in the form of prejudice, patronizing attitudes, and still at other times, it is the result of indifference (Burgdorf & Burgdorf, 1977). Regardless of the origin, the outcomes are the same: exclusion, segregation, or the denial of equal, effective, and meaningful opportunities to participate in activities and programs (Brothwell and Sandison, 1967). The goal of the ADA is preventing and correcting the numerous problems associated with discrimination against people with disabilities (Pardeck & Chung, 1992). A basic social work strategy, advocacy, can be effective as a means for ensuring that the ADA is implemented appropriately (Pardeck, 1998).

The goals of advocacy are to achieve social justice and to empower people. Advocacy helps people correct those situations that are unjust. It requires the active participation of citizens who are vulnerable or disenfranchised; the professional social worker also plays a critical role in this process. The banding together of those who wish to achieve social justice provides the opportunity for empowerment, for active, responsible participation in the public realm (Lewis, 1992). When clients' rights have been denied, the role of the advocate is to speak on behalf of them and to empower clients to speak on their own behalves. The advocacy role is a critical strategy for those who are grounded in a social justice approach to practice because it expands opportunities by protecting the interests of clients. Furthermore, advocacy is a classic role aimed at changing the oppressive social environments of clients, including the various systems that prevent individual growth and development (Pardeck, 1998).

According to McGowan (1987), advocacy can be conducted at two levels, case advocacy and cause advocacy. The case advocacy approach focuses on individual cases. It involves the partisan intervention on behalf of a client or identified client group with one or more secondary institutions to secure or enhance needed services, resources, or entitlements (McGowan, 1987). Cause advocacy seeks to redress collective issues through social change efforts and improving social policies (Pardeck, 1998).

Rees (1991) argues that case and cause advocacy both begin by identifying the dynamics causing social injustice and makes the following conclusion about the advocacy process:

> The decision to pursue the advocacy of a case or a cause, or a combination of both, will usually have been preceded by the identification of an injustice which it is felt cannot be rectified simply by efficient administration or negotiation. The identification of an injustice and the sense of conviction concerning the removal of this injustice should become a priority . . . It is not sufficient merely to recognize an injustice. You have to believe that this issue should be fought for and if necessary over a long period of time. (p. 146)

Miley, O'Melia, and DuBois (1995) conclude that the following issues must be an integral part of the advocacy process aimed at social injustice and social change:

1. The location of the problem must be identified. It must be determined, for example, whether the problem reflects a personal need, a gap in services, or inequitable social policy.
2. The objectives of intervention must be identified. For instance, objectives might be defined as procuring entitlements for clients or expanding job opportunities for oppressed individuals.
3. The target system of advocacy intervention must be identified. This at times might be the practitioner's own agency or other systems the agency works with.
4. The advocate must determine what authority or sanction he or she has to intervene in a targeted system. This can include legal rights of clients and judicial decisions.
5. The resources available for advocacy efforts must be identified. These resources include professional expertise, political influence, and one's credibility and reputation.
6. It must be determined by those involved in an advocacy effort the degree to which the target system is receptive to the proposed advocacy effort. The target system will make this decision based on the reasonableness or lawfulness of the advocacy effort.

7. The level at which the intervention will occur must be analyzed to insure that the desired outcomes will be achieved. Different levels of intervention might include policy changes, modification of administrative procedures, and alterations in the discretionary actions taken by staff or management in an agency.
8. The object of intervention must be identified. This might include individual delivery services, agency administrators, or even a legislative body.
9. The strategies of advocacy intervention must be determined. These strategies include the roles of negotiator, collaborator, and adversary.
10. Those involved in advocacy efforts must learn from the outcomes of prior advocacy efforts, including both failures and successes.

Those who are involved in advocacy efforts must understand the need for this type of intervention with the various systems they work with (Pardeck, 1998). What must be understood, if one considers the plight of people with disabilities, is that public and private entities did not, for example, ask for the passage of the Americans With Disabilities Act. Most of these systems, including schools and businesses, would prefer self-regulation over a federal mandate aimed at protecting people with disabilities. Advocates find that self-regulation does not work and that even after the passage of legislation such as the Americans With Disabilities Act, social systems mandated to conform to this new disability law will attempt to avoid their legal obligations. This means advocacy is an absolute necessity to insure laws, such as the Americans With Disabilities Act, are implemented appropriately (Pardeck, 1998).

There are a number of reasons why entities legally bound by the mandates of civil rights legislation such as the ADA attempt to avoid compliance. First, organizations including schools and private businesses have been provided the compliance materials for the Americans With Disabilities Act; however, because they may contradict the bureaucratic rules of these systems, they often do not follow procedures set forth in compliance materials. The person with a disability brings a unique set of needs to the workplace, including the need at times for reasonable accommodations. Bureaucratic organizations are often rigid systems and are not prone to make exceptions; they literally must be forced to make exceptions through strong advocacy efforts (Pardeck, 1998).

Second, all public and private entities bound by the mandates of the ADA feel that they operate on limited resources. The organization thinks there is an added cost when an employee with a disability requests a reasonable accommodation in order to do his or her job. Organizations asked to provide special accommodations for people with disabilities must be convinced by advocates that this is a requirement of the law, and that the federal mandate for providing reasonable accommodations is based on the needs of the person with a disability and not necessarily on the needs of the organization's budget (Pardeck, 1998).

Third, people are often intimidated by both public and private bureaucracies. A person with a disability may have limited experience and exposure in dealing with organizations in general. Such persons need the help of an expert, the advocate, in dealing with complex organizations. Skillful advocates understand how complex organizations work and are well aware of the regulations these systems must follow, including disability laws (Pardeck, 1998).

Lastly, often it is difficult for persons with disabilities to look at their own problems without their emotions impacting their objectivity. Skillful advocates are able to step back from situations that negatively impact persons with disabilities and provide reason and objectivity to the process for both the person with a disability and the entity who is not complying with the ADA (Pardeck, 1998).

With the ADA as an example, the importance of advocacy even after a law has been passed to protect a category of people becomes clear. Advocacy is about influence and power, ingredients that are often critical to forcing entities to conform to regulations and laws (Pardeck, 1998).

EFFECTIVE ADVOCACY SKILLS FOR PERSONS WITH DISABILITIES

The ADA and other disability laws were enacted to protect the rights of people with disabilities; the history of the ADA suggests that persons with disabilities played a critical role in the creation of this law (Pardeck and Chung, 1992). People with disabilities have a primary responsibility for ensuring that their rights are met under the mandates of the ADA. This can only be achieved if persons with disabilities learn how to effectively advocate on their own behalves. The following strategies and skills are designed to help persons with disabilities become effective advocates for themselves. The goals of the following are to empower persons with disabilities to achieve social justice for themselves and others with disabilities (Pardeck, 1998).

Believing in Their Rights

Persons with disabilities must be taught that they are equal partners with others, such as professional social workers. Equal partnership also means that a person with a disability must accept his or her share of responsibility for solving problems related to advocacy efforts.

Having a Clear Vision

Persons with disabilities must learn to be optimistic and communicate clearly with systems that are denying them their rights under the ADA. While trying to achieve what is perceived as ideal, they must be able to recognize what is realistic.

Organization

Persons with disabilities must be taught to understand that being organized is an absolute necessity to effective advocacy. They must know how to file information, keep track of records, and organize important documentation critical to the advocacy process.

Prioritizing

Persons with disabilities must develop skills in learning how to decide what the most important issues are related to their advocacy efforts. This should be based on their greatest needs as a person with a disability.

Understanding One's Disabilities

A person with a disability must learn everything possible about his or her disability. It is important to acquire indepth information about one's own medical needs, as well as the various assistive technologies available to one as possible reasonable accommodations in the workplace or other settings. This information may help in the resolution of the problem between the person with a disability and an unresponsive system.

Knowing the Law

Persons with disabilities must learn about their rights under the ADA. They also should become familiar with their rights under other federal disability laws.

Following the Chain of Command

It is important for a person with a disability to know that effective advocacy means he or she should first engage those persons that can correct a problem at the lower levels of an organization. If results cannot be obtained at a lower level, then the individual with a disability must move systematically up the chain of command.

Being Informative

The person with a disability must understand his or her special needs and be able to convey all relevant information about his or her disability to the system that advocacy efforts are aimed at. This strategy can be helpful in resolving the problem between the person with a disability and the system denying the person's rights under the ADA.

Offering Solutions

The person with a disability needs to be creative in finding solutions to problems that call for advocacy efforts. Positive solutions are those that benefit everyone involved in the advocacy process.

Being Principled and Persistent

It is important for a person with a disability to master the art of being clear to officials about needed changes. One must keep at the advocacy process and not let the battle become the issue. The person with a disability must avoid being adversarial and realize that he or she must be assertive and not aggressive. One must have a vision that the issue will be resolved to his or her satisfaction.

Learning to Communicate Effectively

A person with a disability must understand that many problems result from poor communication between parties. It is important to learn to listen to what others are saying and to realize that others may have valuable insights into a confronting problem. If a person with a disability does not understand something, he or she must ask questions. It is important to be sincere and honest, and say what is really meant.

Letting Others Know When Pleased

It is important to let the system that has changed because of advocacy efforts hear the person's satisfaction and excitement as the system continues to progress in the area of ADA rights. This kind of positive behavior will help to keep the organization on the right track in the area of disability law.

Developing Endurance

One of the first lessons learned from doing advocacy is that it is important to learn to develop endurance. Advocacy is a process that often extends over a long time period. The person with a disability will face many challenges and issues; some successes and some failures need to be expected. It is important to learn lessons from both.

Following Through

One must make a concerted effort to monitor the process concerning what has been agreed to as a result of the advocacy process. The person with a disability must make sure the accommodation or program changes are being provided appropriately. If the need for a different accommodation emerges, it is critical to advocate for these changes.

Having a Sense of Humor

Advocacy is about endurance. Developing and cultivating a sense of humor is one of the most important traits a person with a disability needs for successful advocacy.

CONCLUSIONS

The authors have overviewed the key components of the ADA. A discussion was offered on why and how persons with disabilities are discriminated against. Critical United States Supreme Court decisions were presented; many of these decisions have greatly limited the power of the ADA in protecting the rights of persons with disabilities. Even though the United States Supreme Court has narrowed the impact of the ADA in American life, a number of EEOC cases were presented in the paper which suggests this federal agency is attempting to protect persons with disabilities against discrimination. The final area covered in the paper dealt with the topic of advocacy; advocacy may well be one of the most effective tools to help insure that the rights of people with disabilities are protected.

The ADA is the most important civil rights law for persons with disabilities. Even though many of the initial intentions of the ADA have been negated by the United States Supreme Court, countless people with disabilities have benefited from the protections of the ADA. It is critical at this time that the United States Congress pass legislation that corrects the attacks on the ADA by the Court. Persons with disabilities need to be advocates for these changes in the legislative process.

REFERENCES

Albertsons, Inc. vs. Kirkingburg (1998), 143 F.3d 1228. *Americans With Disabilities Act of 1989 (The).* (1989). Washington, DC: Government Printing Office.
Americans With Disabilities Act of 1990 (The). (1990). P. L. 101-336, 105 Stat. 327, 42 U.S.C., 12101 et seq.
Arnold, K. (1999). Americans With Disabilities Act: Do cancer patients qualify as disabled? *Journal of the National Cancer Institute, 91*, 822-825.
Board of Trustees of the University of Alabama vs. Garrett (2001). (99-1240) 193 F.3d 1214, reversed.
Bragdon vs. Abbott (1998). 107 F.3d 934.
Brothwell, D. S., & Sandison, A. T. (1967). *Diseases in antiquity.* Springfield, IL: Charles C. Thomas.
Burgdorf, R. L., & Burgdorf, M. P. (1977). The wicked witch is almost dead: Buck vs. Bell and the sterilization of handicapped persons. *Temple Law Quarterly, 50*, 995-1054.
Castro, I. L. (2000). *A report on the tenth anniversary of the Americans With Disabilities Act (ADA).* http://www.eeoc.gov/ ada/statusreport.html
Cleveland vs. Policy Management (1997). 120 F.3d 513.
Equal Employment Opportunity Commission & U. S. Department of Justice (1992). The Americans With Disabilities Act: Questions and answers. Washington, DC: National Institute on Disabilities and Rehabilitation Research.
Federal Register (1980). No. 66. Washington, DC: U. S. Printing.
Harrison, M., & Gilbert, S. (Eds.) (1992). *The Americans With Disabilities Act handbook.* Beverly Hills, CA: Excellent Books.
Ianacone, B.P. (1977). Historical overview: From charity to rights. *Temple Law Quarterly 50*: 953-960.
Lewis, E. (1992). Social change and citizen action: A philosophical exploration for modern social group work. *Social Work With Groups, 14*, 23-34.
McGowan, B. G. (1987). Advocacy. In A. Minahan (Ed.), *Encyclopedia of social work: Vol. 1* (18th ed., pp. 89-95). Silver Spring, MD: National Association of Social Workers.
Miley, K. K., O'Melia, M., & DuBois, B. (1995). *Generalist social work practice: An empowering approach.* Boston: Allyn and Bacon.
Murphy vs. United Parcel Service Inc. (1998). 141 F.3d 1185.
Olmstead vs. L.C. (1998). 138 F3d 893.

Pardeck, J. T. (1998). *Social work after the Americans With Disabilities Act: New challenges and opportunities for social service professionals.* Westport: CT: Auburn House.

Pardeck, J. T. (2001). An update on the Americans With Disabilities Act: Implications for health and human services delivery. *Journal of Health and Social Policy, 13,* 1-15.

Pardeck, J. T. (2002a). An overview and comments on recent Americans With Disabilities Act court rulings. *Journal of Social Work in Disability and Rehabilitation, 1*(1), 5-14.

Pardeck, J. T. (2002b). Knowledge, tasks, and strategies for teaching about persons with disabilities: Implications for social work education. *Journal of Social Work in Disability and Rehabilitation, 1*(2), 53-72.

Pardeck, J. T., & Chung, W. (1992). An analysis of the Americans With Disabilities Act of 1990. *Journal of Health and Social Policy, 4,* 47-56.

Pennsylvania Department of Corrections vs. Yeskey (1997). 118 F.3d 168.

Rees, S. (1991). *Achieving power: Practice and policy in social welfare.* North Sydney, Australia: Allen & Unwin.

Sutton vs. United Airlines (1997). 130 F.3d 893.

doi:10.1300/J198v06n01_05

Planned Change in the Disability Community

Randall R. Myers

SUMMARY. Planned change with people, who are physically or mentally disabled, as with other special populations, requires a range of skills and knowledge; several specific aspects of the change process are identified and discussed in this article: the characteristics of the change agent, the timing of the change event, and creating a vision for change. These aspects are illustrated through the writer's own experiences as a change agent working a long-range change event to improve access[1] to mental health services in the US with and for people who are deaf and hard of hearing. doi:10.1300/J198v06n01_06 *[Article copies available for a fee from The Haworth Document Delivery Service: 1-800-HAWORTH. E-mail address: <docdelivery@haworthpress.com> Website: <http://www.HaworthPress.com> © 2007 by The Haworth Press, Inc. All rights reserved.]*

KEYWORDS. Change agent, deaf/hard of hearing, planned change, physical and mental disability, standards of care

INTRODUCTION

Over the past 50 years or more, there has been an increasing and dramatic proliferation of planned change efforts on behalf of the 54 million people (National Organization On Disability website, 2004) who have

Randall R. Myers, PhD, LCSW-C, is Consultant, RRMyers Consulting, 3905 Blackburn Lane, # 24, Burtonsville, MD 20866 (E-mail: rrmyers@comcast.net).

[Haworth co-indexing entry note]: "Planned Change in the Disability Community." Myers, Randall R. Co-published simultaneously in *Journal of Social Work in Disability & Rehabilitation* (The Haworth Press, Inc.) Vol. 6, No. 1/2, 2007, pp. 93-109; and: *Disability and Social Work Education: Practice and Policy Issues* (ed: Francis K. O. Yuen, Carol B. Cohen, and Kristine Tower) The Haworth Press, Inc., 2007, pp. 93-109. Single or multiple copies of this article are available for a fee from The Haworth Document Delivery Service [1-800-HAWORTH, 9:00 a.m. - 5:00 p.m. (EST). E-mail address: docdelivery@haworthpress.com].

physical, developmental, and mental disabilities in the US. These initiatives have resulted in an emerging disability policy framework (Silverstein, 2000) focusing on building access[1] to many of society's activities and advantages and affecting all spheres of life. The activities and advantages of these Federal policies have been more tangible in nature, such as *architecture* through the Architectural Barriers Act of 1968 (P.L. 90-480), *transportation* through the Federal–Aid Highway Act of 1973 (P.L. 93-87), *technology* through the Assistive Technology Act of 1998 (P.L.105-394), and *telecommunications* through the Telecommunications Act of 1996 (P.L.104-104). Others have been in a sense more intangible, such as *education* through the Education for All Handicapped Children (P.L. 94-142) in 1975, Developmental Disabilities Assistance and Bill of Rights Act (P.L. 94-103) in 1975, and Protection and Advocacy for Mentally Ill Individuals Act of 1986 (P.L. 99-319). These policies culminated, of course, in the Americans With Disabilities Act (P.L. 101-336) in 1990. Each of these federal policies has their concomitant policy at the state and local levels, so that change is not limited to taking place on the Federal level or only in Federal level institutions. These efforts have focused on changes in a wide range of large systems and institutions, such as universities and colleges, state government departments, and even corporate change in the private sector. A multitude of planned change efforts bring the impact of this legislation to more local levels–ultimately to counties, communities, agencies, programs, and services.

　　Most, if not all, of these efforts follow from the civil rights movement, originating in the 1960's in the United States and concluding with the passage of Title VI of the Civil Rights Act of 1964 and have been spearheaded by individuals or groups: private citizens, family members, professionals, legislators, and innumerable different kinds of groups in different spheres of society. These groups may be labeled as task forces, coalitions, partnerships, associations, and alliances, just to name a few. For example, the signing of the Americans With Disabilities Act in 1990 was preceded by an intense flurry of disability community lobbying from 1988 to 1990. This lobby was "organizing and galvanizing policy advocates in and out of Congress" (Watson, 1993, p. 31). Watson notes that these advocates included legislators with personal motivations and three types of coalitions concerned with different disabilities and primary interests: (1) Individuals with different kinds of disabilities; (2) Groups with no past affiliation with the cause; and (3) Political figures with a broad, bipartisan range of experience and interest in disability rights.

"Given the seemingly natural propensity of some service systems to be insensitive to the needs of special populations, individuals and groups have recognized increasingly that it is in their interest to organize for collective action. Collective power is a means for effecting change in the way human service programs are conceptualized, designed, and delivered. Groups have organized around common concerns and needs related to age, race, gender, sexual preference, marital status, handicapping condition, and many other characteristics. Formally organized groups have developed and used political, economic, and legal power to ensure attention to special needs and concerns. Funding requirements, policy guidelines, and legal precedents have established the rights of designated target populations to services"(Kettner, Daley, & Nichols, 1985, p. 3).

From the broader view, to be sure, collective action has promoted growing awareness and stimulated change, but there are many, many individuals within these organizing groups who help to mobilize and carry out planned change in general and collectively-agreed-upon direction. Mackelprang and Salsgiver (1996) note, however, that the social work profession has not done much to serve people with disabilities nor done much to advance disability rights. There also few social workers with disabilities working in the field. This, however, is changing as public and professional sensitivity and demand for access increase. Nevertheless, one day you may be a social worker, whether you have a disabling condition or not, who will be in a position of working on some aspect of change for the Disability community. Somewhere, sometime, somehow, you may be in a service delivery system that should be serving and/or being accessible to people who are *physically, mentally, culturally,* or *linguistically* diverse. And you may be in a position to help.

The goal of this article is to sensitize social work students to joining with the broader Disability community for macro intervention change specifically of, by, and for people who are disabled–for the student to be aware of their role and function as social workers in a change event when working with this very diverse population. This article does not purport to cover every aspect of what is known or needed for social work macro interventions, but only to direct attention to several critical aspects that are salient for serving this population. Accordingly, this article briefly defines disability and then addresses characteristics of the change agent, the timing of the change effort, and sharing a vision for change.

Throughout this article, the development of the *Standards of Care for the Delivery of Mental Health Services to Deaf and Hard of Hearing Persons* from 1990 to 1995 will be used as an example of a long-range social work macro intervention with people who have a hearing loss. As the reader may or may not be familiar, this particular disability population has special needs related to their culture, communication, and language to achieve equal access to mental health and substance abuse services and, indeed, most of what society has to offer. After the idea of creating practice guidelines was floated among specialized practitioners in the mid-1980's, this writer has been the change agent for that particular mental health initiative since 1992 to the present; some aspects of my profile as a change agent and my experience will be noted. In addition, the history of the development of mental health services for this population in the US may also be instructive to the reader about how a combination of various professionals, organizations, funding, and support presented the ideal conditions, i.e., the context for the development of such a milestone document and indications for the possibility of significant change in mental health system access for this population.

WHAT IS DISABILITY?

Disability can be defined from a *psychological* perspective, i.e., the interplay between personality development and physical and mental limitations; as an *economic* phenomenon viewing disability as a product of income and social position; as a *sociological* function of how institutions (families, schools, hospitals, etc.) treat people with physical and mental limitations; as a *political* division or category that explores how disability is shaped through the institutions of government (Stone, 1984), or as a legal phenomenon (Minow, 1990).

In the context of this chapter, disability is defined consistent with the mission and values of the Society for Disability Studies (SDS): Disability is viewed as a social construction shaped by various institutions and systems, but primarily as a key aspect of human experience on par with race, class, gender, sex, and sexual orientation. Disability is the result of personal and collective responses to difference. I suggest that disability can be viewed as 'difference,' whether that difference is physical, mental, cultural, or linguistic.

CHARACTERISTICS OF THE CHANGE AGENT

There are a number of social welfare change efforts we are all familiar with and see on a day-to-day basis, often initiated by highly visible individuals who point to a particular issue and say, "The public needs to be sensitized to what is happening" or "This or that needs to be changed," for example, Michael Moore who produced the movie *Bowling for Columbine* (2002) about the dangers of firearm possession in America and Morgan Spurlock's film, *Supersize Me!* (2004), raising awareness about personal and corporate responsibility for obesity in the US. These are global efforts to focus public attention on a critical social problem led by one highly visible individual or producer, but they give us a good hint of what we need to know in order to make change: there will be a group of consumers of service and many stakeholders with differing interests and values.

First we focus on the characteristics of the change agent. Wertheimer, (2003) asks:

What types of individuals can mobilize a system to change? What are the specific skills required to promote integration across multiple systems? Where in the system should the change agent be placed? The answers to these questions may help to ensure that integration efforts produce long-term solutions to significant system problems through a process that preserves dignity and respect for both consumers of services and the full range of stakeholders across multiple systems. True change agents must be comfortable assuming different roles at different times. Sometimes the change agent needs to address the seemingly endless obstacles to change that are contained within various statutory, regulatory and even clinical environments. (p. 1)

Change Agent in the Deaf community–Personal Aspects

As a hearing child of deaf parents, I had the opportunity to become fluent in American Sign Language, embrace Deaf culture, and internalize a visual communication process at a very early age. I have been able to use and apply this extensive knowledge, skill, and experience to the change process even though I do not have a hearing loss myself.

Although I had these requisite skills and knowledge, I needed to gain the confidence of people in the Deaf community and in the general social work/mental health field in order to be effective as a change agent. As a licensed clinician with a masters in social work degree, I began counseling deaf and hard of hearing consumers and learning about their experiences and frustrations accessing mental health services. I was also able to observe how states, programs, and service providers addressed access challenges for this population, how these approaches affected service delivery, and the frustrations of my consumers and colleagues who were receiving and providing direct care services various social work settings.

After providing outpatient counseling services, where could I go to begin my career as a change agent advocate? The State appeared to be the best, most accessible, setting to effect change–where I could learn how the system worked from the inside.

Fluency in the language, culture, and communication process of the people you are working with definitely facilitate the goals for change, but somehow I believe they are not the essential elements. The illustration, above, suggests that the essential elements lean more towards (1) sensitivity and opportunity for individual access choice(s); (2) knowledge of resources for access; and (3) how the system operates in terms of approach to access for the population being served.

Social work with people who are disabled takes place in all three sectors, public, private, and non-profit on all levels of government and community service. Services are provided to people who are disabled in a multitude of milieu, such as health, education, legal, and criminal justice. Diagram 1 conceptualizes how human services are provided

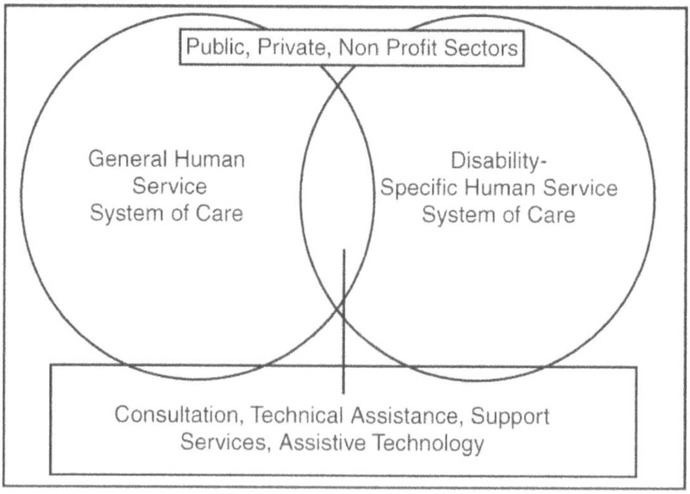

DIAGRAM 1. Human Service System Access to Competent System of Care

in environments exclusively geared for people who are disabled and in the general human service milieu and how they overlap.

HUMAN SERVICE SYSTEM ACCESS
TO COMPETENT SYSTEM OF CARE

A variety of communication and cultural brokers, facilitators, or technology may be used to ensure communication of access choice at some level of confidence and effectiveness. I realized that services and programs provided or funded by large organizations, however intentional or inadvertent, often deny opportunity for consumer participation on an even "playing field;" human service organizations and programs often need to make concerted and directed efforts to redesign, reconfigure, or redirect programs, policies, and procedures to meet the access needs of special population consumers with special needs.

An example of this for people with mental disabilities is Curie's recent Substance Abuse and Mental Health Administration's statement (Curie, 2004) about mental health recovery, "Increasingly, people coping with mental and addictive disorders are redefining the meaning of recovery. Historically, recovery has been regarded as abstinence from drugs or the absence of symptoms. But emerging definitions seek to go beyond abstinence or absence to include re-engagement with life.

At SAMHSA, our vision is of a life in the community for everyone–a fulfilling life that includes a job, a home, and meaningful relationships with family and friends. Our mission is to make this vision a reality, by building resilience and facilitating recovery for people with substance abuse and mental illness.

Our vision and our mission guide all our efforts here at SAMHSA: our policies and programs. So it makes sense to evaluate the outcomes of our programs within the context of recovery" (p. 3).

Mr. Curie is a social worker by profession and announced a major change in his agency's direction by building into the agency's mission the value of recovery in policy and programming. How this change comes about is related to timing–the opportunity for change presents in various ways and it is incumbent on the social worker to seize these opportunities; this might appear somewhat abstract, but as will be shown in the next section of this chapter, there are several indicators that, if observed and interpreted correctly, will signal an open door for change.

THE OPPORTUNITY FOR CHANGE–
THE TIMING OF THE CHANGE EFFORT BUILDING
ON HISTORICAL DEVELOPMENTS

The first indicator of the potential for change is historical antecedents. This begins with doing some research and observation regarding existing policy and/or changes that have been made related to the change that needs to occur. Taken together, these events appear to point in the direction of potential change and may include legal decisions, research initiatives, and the significant development of new types of services and programs. On a more programmatic level, they might include steps taken to develop mission statements and agency policy and procedures. Using mental health services provided to people who are deaf or hard of hearing, here is an example of several historical antecedents that indicate the potential of improved access to mental health services for this population.

DEVELOPMENT OF MENTAL HEALTH SERVICES
FOR PEOPLE WHO ARE DEAF OR HARD OF HEARING

Coordinated service delivery for this population begins in the mid to late 1950s with the establishment of two specialized inpatient units for research and treatment in New York and Washington, D.C. (Rockland State and St. Elizabeth's Hospitals, respectively) through the efforts of Rainer, Altshuler, and Robinson, three respected psychiatrists. These inpatient units were funded through a special grant from the Federal Department of Health, Education, and Welfare (HEW) that no longer exists and is now named the Department of Health and Human Services. Prior to these events, services were provided primarily through the fields of vocational rehabilitation and education (Vernon, 1995; Pollard, 1992-93). Subsequently, opportunities for more advanced learning, hands-on experience, and employment were made available in the field especially for professionals who were deaf or hard of hearing themselves and/or fluent signers. In addition, the National Association of the Deaf had a Mental Health Committee made up of many of these trained professionals who were, themselves, deaf or hard of hearing. In the late '70s, this committee strongly recommended the creation of a "Model State Plan" since . . . "a vast majority of states do not provide specialized mental health services . . . and . . . current guidelines and regulations . . . are not applicable to the special needs . . ." of this population (Scanlan, 1978, p. 67).

Following these initial events, mental health service and program development expanded rapidly across the United States, buoyed by the Americans With Disabilities Act of 1990 (ADA), and paved the way for the development of a standards of care for this population.

Alignment of Stakeholders

A second critical indicator of change potential is how stakeholders are thinking about a specific issue for their disability concern. Within the Disability community as with any other, there are government agencies, such as the National Council on Disability (www.ncd.gov); the National Organization on Disability (www.nod.com) whose mission is to expand the contribution and participation of people with disabilities throughout society; the American Association of People with Disabilities, AAPD, that is "the largest national nonprofit cross-disability member organization in the United States, dedicated to ensuring economic self-sufficiency and political empowerment for the more than 56 million Americans with disabilities" (AAPD website www.aapd.org); organizations that support and foster academic and research on disability, for example, the Society for Disability Studies (SDS); organizations that focus on resources, for example, the National Dissemination Center for Children with Disabilities (NICHCY); National Alliance for the Mentally Ill, ". . . a nonprofit, grassroots, self-help, support and advocacy organization of consumers, families, and friends of people with severe mental illnesses . . ." (NAMI website: www.nami.org), and a multitude of commissions, committees, task forces, throughout the states that advocate for improved conditions for people with disabilities. There are organizations that serve the general Disability community and others that serve specific physical, mental, or developmental disability groups.

Some change initiatives will only involve a specific disability group and others will cross disability concerns. Regardless, the beginning of any change attempt focuses first on knowing and working to shape the disposition of those within the particular disability group. McGuire (1993) describes in her article how "tenuous" and, at the same time, "resilient" was the solidarity of the Disability community advocating up to the passage of the ADA and the two legislative bills that preceded it. The passage of the ADA was truly a remarkable achievement!

Deaf Community Support for Access

In the previous insert above, I noted that the National Association of the Deaf (NAD) and mental health professionals serving people who are deaf or hard of hearing had clearly indicated support for changes in mental health access for this population. In addition, several Deaf communities in various states across the country were now taking independent action in terms of advocating for specialized programming and services and sometimes enlisting the legal system through lawsuits and consent decrees. In the early '90s, ADARA (American Deafness and Rehabilitation Association), a non-profit organization serving human service professionals who work with people who are deaf and hard of hearing, initiated the development of a "Model State Mental Health Plan" through a subcommittee headed up by Paul Loera, PhD, from Pittsburgh, PA. Later on in the development of the Model State Plan (later renamed the "Standards of Care"), there would need to be an effort in the future to broaden the appeal and value of such a document *within both organizations*, but the establishment of an ADARA committee was a good beginning.

Sharing a Vision for Change

Creating a vision for change is a critical aspect of social work macro intervention work since everyone involved needs to work towards common goals and be clear as to what those goals are. The presentation and creation of vision can, potentially, take place at many different times and for different reasons during the life of a change event or various episodes while change is developing or taking place.

To begin with, any group of individuals, for example people who are disabled, must first use their collective power of reflection to realize their situation, or the situation that they find themselves in, before they can visualize a way out (Mondros and Wilson, 1994; Pecukonis and Wenocur, 1994; Rothman, 1974; Freire, 1970; Memmi, 1965). They have to be able to somehow see that their *situation* as not satisfactory and be able to see it differently, "Functionally, oppression is domesticating. To no longer be prey to its force, one must emerge from it and turn upon it. This can be done only by means of the praxis: reflection and action upon the world in order to transform it" (Freire, 1970, p. 36).

Following reflection, the creation of a vision helps build *confidence* that the process of change will happen and that it is the right thing to do and *competence*, including skill building, to actually carry out and be involved in the change process.

The Well-Placed Change Agent

In 1989, my previous personal and professional experiences (noted earlier in this article) worked together with my new administrative position to solidify my role as a potentially well-placed change agent. I was able to closely observe system operations first-hand in my new position as Deaf State Program Coordinator in the (then) Illinois Department of Mental Health and Developmental Disabilities (IDMHDD). These events were well-timed with ADARA's fledgling efforts to develop a model state plan. As State Coordinator, I was able to develop ". . . an understanding of some basic principles of organizational structure and function. Studying the rationale for hierarchy, authority, formal lines of communication, job descriptions, written job qualifications, clearly defined policies and procedures, and formal procedures for personnel selection, training, and development . . ." (Kettner, Daley, and Nichols, 1985, p. 14) helped me understand the inner workings of large public sector organizations, in this case, a state department of mental health. Most important, along with the Deaf community, I saw what needed to change: The system needed to be more responsive, through policy, procedures, and services, to making mental health services more accessible for people who are deaf or hard of hearing.

"Shared perceptions" (Pecukonis and Wenocur, 1994, p. 13) or a vision of what can be serve to strengthen hopefulness and self-efficacy (Bandura, 1977) particularly in the collective, e.g., groups or social action organizations. Some visions that advocate for immediate, and others for more long-term, change, can be communicated many ways. We have seen several in our lifetimes: marches, demonstrations, written papers, and other consciousness-raising media. Some visions or shared perceptions are more overt and others are more subtle in dissemination and long-term impact.

Building and Sharing the Vision: Defining Specialized Services

Two essential aspects of building a shared perception or a vision for planned change are (1) defining and being clear about the access elements that are unique to a specific disability. A good deal of research and observation is needed to achieve clear definition, for example, through interviews and information from a variety of sources, such as organization newsletters, research studies, journal articles, consumer anecdotal reports, and media. (2) establishing connections with allies, i.e., identifying individuals (also known as *key stakeholders*) who support these access elements and agree with a vision of improved access being proposed and by establishing a *coalition*. Stakeholders and coalitions can include anyone, for example, family members, consumers, professional service providers, legislators, and organization and program staff.

In the field of mental health, for example, the delivery of quality and competent services for children depends on an appropriate and competent mental health assessment for services or referral to receive appropriate care (National Council on Disability, 2002). A planned macro intervention to improve this delivery system might use the diagram, presented earlier, to visualize two overlapping systems of care that reflect a general mental health system on the left and services specifically modified or structured for a specific disability group, for example, children with severe emotional disturbances. For all of these children, service delivery access considers, for example, mental health service access for families or alternative living situations, educators, and transition to work and adulthood. How might the needs of these children be met in the traditional school milieu and what ancillary or additional services might they need to meet these needs?

DEFINING SPECIALIZED MENTAL HEALTH SERVICES FOR PEOPLE WHO ARE DEAF OR HARD OF HEARING

People with hearing loss continually struggle with communication access in everyday life and on a daily basis. Since mental health services rely heavily on the expression of self, confidentiality, and language skill to facilitate individual change, access to mental health, substance abuse and developmental disability services can be particularly challenging for this population.

The *Standards of Care* (Myers, 1995) proposes a model for assessing an individual with hearing loss' cultural and communication needs that includes referral to a "level of access" within any particular treatment milieu for appropriate care. These access levels, in essence, reflect increasing cultural competence skills when working with this population. In other words, depending on an individual's choice(s), cultural affiliation, and communication skills, a deaf, hard of hearing, late deafened, or deafblind person may *choose* to receive services in a cross-cultural *or* cultural milieu. For example, a Deaf person who signs may be more inclined to request a therapist who also signs. A person who has some hearing, or who is hard of hearing, may prefer a provider who can empathize with their client's hearing loss and who is aware of the technological resources available, for example, hearing aids or assistive listening devices.

Building and Sharing the Vision:
Involving Stakeholders in the Change Process

Stakeholders are involved in a planned change event for the purpose of encouraging or advocating for the proposed change (the shared vision) to happen, but also to help build and share the vision among their respective constituencies. The change agent orchestrates planned change events largely through the work of stakeholders. Each stakeholder joins the coalition and is able to contribute their individual strengths and contacts to the effort. Continuing with the example of children who have severe emotional disturbances, perhaps the change agent might be in a position to meet with several parents or attend a PTA meeting or communicate with a few mental health providers to identify some improvements that might be made to support the emotional needs of these children in school. Initially these individuals might identify common concerns and then, as a group, formulate the kind of change they would like to see happen. Each stakeholder would explore these changes in their own groups, for example, the parents might bring up the issue at a PTA meeting and then report back to the coalition. During this period, a great deal of information and background will be obtained that will influence how and whether change can occur. From that point, if a common vision can be agreed upon for change within the coalition, more specific plans and a strategy may be developed to pursue the change effort further.

Making Connections:
Opportunity Knocks

As Illinois' Deaf State Program Coordinator in 1990, I met the (then) Executive Director of the National Association of State Mental Health Program Directors (NASMHPD), Harry Schnibbe, at a state research conference and asked if his organization could do a nationwide survey of State Deaf Services. Then, as a member of ADARA, I read about the Model State Plan Committee and asked in 1992 if I could join and be part of its creation. I brought this NASMHPD information, i.e., what was happening in the states, to the committee meeting in 1992 and proposed a vision for the Model State Plan. The vision included the idea of further defining and promoting specialized services for this population and some ideas about how the Model State Plan document could be used. As shown earlier in the historical reviews, the concept of specialized Deaf Services had been handed down over the years (Sussman, 1990; Galloway, 1969), were the shared perceptions of Deaf community members and the professionals who provided specialized services, but had never been defined or documented in any systematic way. The Model State Plan, now had a more general title of Standards of Care for the Delivery of Mental Health Services to Deaf and Hard of Hearing Persons or *Standards of Care (SOC)* for short.

The Standards of Care were developed from 1992 to 1995 primarily through the work of over 50 culturally and linguistically competent professionals. The first steps of development focused on ensuring that there existed Deaf community anecdotal reports and statements of support for the idea and initiative of creating a model state plan or standards of care. These anecdotes and statements of support would help generate and draw together consensus from the professional community of people who provide mental health and substance abuse services to this population. It would also solidify an alliance between these two key stakeholders. This was accomplished through an intensive literature review and draft reification process at Deaf community and professional national and local conferences to ensure broad consensus, opinion, and clear definition of culturally and linguistically-affirmative access. A State Coordinator conference was held in 1994 with the National Association of State Mental Health Program Directors and several other key stakeholders to bring the Standards of Care to state departments of mental health, another key stakeholder.

It was important for stakeholders to understand how the Standards of Care might help them in their work by: acting as a repository for relevant policies, rules, procedures, and resources.

- helping to build on existing services towards the most needed and possible improvements in various situations;
- functioning as a policy and planning tool providing a framework for discussion and planning with allies;
- providing a comparative basis for assessing the unmet needs of consumers in the community; and

• making the case for culturally and linguistically affirmative mental health policies and programs (Myers, 1998).

CONCLUSION

This article discussed several key factors to creating planned change, specifically the characteristics of the change agent, the timing of the change effort, and the sharing of a common vision for change.
There are several key concluding points to be made:

> *First, the timing/sequencing of planned change events is critical.* Change agents need to recognize and seize opportunities for change as, perhaps, reflected in historical or background information, anecdotal evidence, or through several data or information sources that may appear to be unrelated. The change agent needs to be able to take advantage of resources and opportunities as they are presented in order to present the vision and promote shared consensus. All of these opportunities must be seen as means towards the same change goal.
>
> *Second, the change process is slow and deliberate.* As the expression goes, "Things do not happen overnight." The pace of the change process allows for a critical ongoing and sustained dialogue to ensue. Stakeholders must have opportunity to talk about the change that they support and get feedback into the process.
>
> *Third, change agent commitment and follow-through are essential* ingredients for a planned change effort. The length of this commitment depends on the scope of the effort.

To work with and on behalf of a special population, like people who are disabled, in the capacity of a change agent is both an honor and a responsibility that cannot be taken lightly. True change depends on honesty and commitment to service. Once the change process has begun, more and more people begin to depend on the changes to come and the availability and access to resources.

ENDNOTES

1. The term "access" may be defined generally or in terms of a specific milieu or venue. In the fields of health and mental health, for example, the concept of access to care is generally defined as the ability to obtain needed care or "those dimensions

which describe the potential and actual entry of a given population group to the health care delivery system" (Aday and Anderson, 1974).

* Standards of Care Document in its entirety may be downloaded at: http://www. deafhoh-health.org/resources/mhstandards/ or purchased through the National Association of the Deaf (www.nad.org)

REFERENCES

Aday, L., & Anderson, R. (1974). A framework for the study of access to medical care. *Health Services Research, 9,* 108-220.

Bandura, A. (1977). Self-efficacy: Towards a unifying theory of behavioral change. *Psychological Review, 84,* 191-215.

Curie, C. G. (2004). The promise of recovery. *SAMHSA News.* September/October 2004, *12*(5).

Freire, P. (1970). *Pedagogy of the oppressed.* New York: Continuum.

Galloway, V. H. (1969). Mental health: What it means to the typical deaf person. In K. Z. Altshuler & J. D. Ranier (Eds.) *Mental health and the deaf: Approaches and prospects,* (pp. 51-61). Washington, DC: US Department of Health, Education, & Welfare.

Glickman, N. S. & Zitter, S. M. (1989). On establishing a culturally affirmative psychiatric inpatient program for deaf people. *Journal of the American Deafness & Rehabilitation Association, 23*(2), 46-59.

Kettner, P. M., Daley, J. M., & Nichols, A. W. (1985). *Initiating change in organizations and communities: A macro practice model.* Monterey, California: Brooks/Cole.

Mackelprang, R.W., and Salsgiver, R. O. (1996). People with disabilities and social work: Historical and contemporary issues. *Social Work, 41*(1), 7-14.

McGuire, J. F. (1993). Organizing from diversity in the name of community: Lessons from the disability civil rights movement. In S. D. Watson & D. Pfeiffer (Eds.). *Symposium on Disability Policy, Part Two: Disability Politics and Practice, Policy Studies Journal, 22*(1), 112-122.

Memmi, A. (1965). *The colonizer and the colonized.* Boston: Beacon Press.

Minow, M. (1990). *Making all the difference: Inclusion, exclusion, and American law.* Ithaca: Cornell University Press.

Mondros, J .B., and Wilson, S. M (1994). *Organizing for power and empowerment.* New York: Columbia University Press.

Myers, R. R. (1993). The model mental health state plan (MMHSP) of services for persons who are deaf or hard of hearing. *Journal of the American Deafness and Rehabilitation Association. 27*(1), 19-28.

Myers, R. R. (1995). *Standards of Care for the Delivery of Mental Health Services to Deaf and Hard of Hearing Persons.* Silver Springs, Maryland: National Association of the Deaf.*

National Council on Disability (2002). The well being of our nation: An inter-generational vision of effective mental health services and supports. Washington, DC: National Council on Disability.

National Organization on Disability (2004). Retrieved January 2, 2005, from http://www.nod.org/about/

Pecukonis, E. V., & Wenocur, S. (1994). Perceptions of self and collective efficacy in community organization theory and practice. *Journal of Community Practice, 1*(2), 5-21.

Pollard, R. (1992-1993). 100 years in psychology and deafness: A centennial retrospective. *Journal of the American Deafness and Rehabilitation Association. 25*(3). 32-46.

Rothman, J. (1974). *Planning and organizing for social change: Action principles from social science research.* New York: Columbia University Press.

Scanlan, J. M. (1978). Letter to Fred Schreiber, Executive Secretary, NAD, May 26, 1978. Re: Meetings of the Committee on Mental Health and Deafness. In Minutes of the 34th Biennial Convention, National Association of the Deaf, July 2-8, 1978, Rochester, New York (pp. 66-68). Silver Spring, MD: National Association of the Deaf.

Silverstein, R. (2000). *Emerging disability policy framework: A guidepost for analyzing public policy.* 83 Iowa L. Rev. 1691 (2000).

Stone, D. A. (1984). *The disabled state.* Philadelphia: Temple University Press.

Sussman, A. (1990). Let the buyer beware: Psychotherapy and the deaf consumer. *Gallaudet Today,* Spring, 22-29.

Vernon, M. (1995) An historical perspective on psychology and deafness. *Journal of the American Deafness and Rehabilitation Association, 29*(2), 8-13.

Watson, S. D. (1993). A study in legislative strategy: The passage of the ADA. In L. Gostin and H. Beyer (Eds.) *The Americans With Disabilities Act: What it means for ALL Americans* (pp. 25-33). Baltimore: Paul H. Brookes.

Wertheimer, D. M., M.S.W., M. Div., (March 2001). *Core Qualities of the Change Agent. NASMHPD TOOL BOX No. 8 in a series.*

doi:10.1300/J198v06n01_06

Integrating a Family-Centered Approach into Social Work Practice with Families of Children and Adolescents with Disabilities

Diana Strock-Lynskey
Diane W. Keller

SUMMARY. This article identifies a family-centered practice construct for working with children and adolescents with disabilities and their families. The experiences of these families have shifted considerably over the past 30 years. A legislative and historical context provides the basis for an understanding of present policies and practices that influence current approaches to service delivery. Though family-centered practice is emphasized in various practice settings, there is still a need to integrate this philosophy into social work practice with children and adolescents with disabilities and their families. In order to enhance the ability of the social worker to integrate this construct into practice, a framework for

---

Diana Strock-Lynskey, Professor, MSW, is Chair and Program Director, Department of Social Work, Sienna College Work House, Loudonville, NY 12211 (E-mail: strock@siena.edu). Diane W. Keller, PhD, LSW, is Associate Professor, School of Social Work, Marywood University, 2300 Adams Avenue, Scranton, PA 18509 (E-mail: keller@marywood.edu).

[Haworth co-indexing entry note]: "Integrating a Family-Centered Approach into Social Work Practice with Families of Children and Adolescents with Disabilities." Strock-Lynskey, Diana, and Diane W. Keller. Co-published simultaneously in *Journal of Social Work in Disability & Rehabilitation* (The Haworth Press, Inc.) Vol. 6, No. 1/2, 2007, pp. 111-134; and: *Disability and Social Work Education: Practice and Policy Issues* (ed: Francis K. O. Yuen, Carol B. Cohen, and Kristine Tower) The Haworth Press, Inc., 2007, pp. 111-134. Single or multiple copies of this article are available for a fee from The Haworth Document Delivery Service [1-800-HAWORTH, 9:00 a.m. - 5:00 p.m. (EST). E-mail address: docdelivery@haworthpress.com].

Available online at http://jswdr.haworthpress.com
doi:10.1300/J198v06n01_07

exploring the experiences of children, adolescents and families is provided. This framework provides an overview of factors related to the individual child, the family and siblings for the social worker to consider
when working with these families. The social worker's role as collaborator, advocate, team member and family resource is highlighted. doi:10.1300/
J198v06n01_07 *[Article copies available for a fee from The Haworth Document Delivery
Service: 1-800-HAWORTH. E-mail address: <docdelivery@haworthpress.com> Website:
<http://www.HaworthPress.com> © 2007 by The Haworth Press, Inc. All rights reserved.]*

KEYWORDS. Children and adolescents, legislation and policy, family
centered approach, culturally diverse families, developmental assets,
intervention strategies

INTRODUCTION

The experiences of families who have children and/or adolescents
with disabilities have shifted considerably over the past 30 years. In
1967, it was estimated that over 200,000 children with mental retardation, mental health conditions, sensory impairments, and health conditions that affected cognitive functioning, physical functioning and/or
mobility (e.g., epilepsy, cerebral palsy, to note a few) grew up and lived
away from their families in state institutions. In the 1960s, schools in
the United States provided public education for only about 20% of children with disabilities, depending on the nature of their condition (U.S.
Department of Education, 2004). This was due to the fact that the majority of children with disabilities, particularly those categorized as "severe" in nature and residing in institutional settings did not receive any
educational or therapeutic services or skills training. [See the collected
papers of Burton Blatt (Taylor & Blatt, 1999) and selected speeches of
Gunnar Dybwad (Allard, Howard, Vorderer & Wells, 1999) for more
in-depth background.]

During the mid to late 60s, the deinstitutionalization, independent
living and consumer advocacy movements served as the catalyst for a
major shift in how children with disabilities began to be viewed. Primarily based on the urging of parents, legislators and federal government officials began to focus more attention on meeting the educational
needs of children with disabilities.

TWENTIETH LEGISLATION AND POLICY PERTAINING DIRECTLY TO CHILDREN WITH DISABILITIES: IMPLICATIONS FOR FAMILIES

In 1966, amendments were made in the Elementary and Secondary Education Act of 1965 authorizing funds to assist states "in the initiation, expansion, and improvement of programs for the education of handicapped children" (DePoy & French Gilson, 2004, p. 36). Eligibility for resources expanded to include school-age children with diagnostic, cognitive, psychiatric and physical conditions.

In 1968, the Handicapped Children's Early Education Assistance Act provided resources to children enrolled in school and pre-school programs and coincided with a landmark shift in stance from legislation focused primarily on the provision of resources to the recognition of civil rights with the passage, in 1968, of the Architectural Barriers Act and the later passage of the Rehabilitation Act of 1973 (DePoy & French Gilson, 2004, p. 35). Section 504 of this act provides civil rights protections to individuals with disabilities with special needs and requires that special rehabilitative services be provided to children while in school (Library of Congress, Thomas on the Internet, 2004).

During the 1970s, stronger emphasis was placed on the rights of individuals with disabilities to be able to exercise self-determination and control over one's own life, including the ability to live as independently as possible within the context of the broader society. Greater pressure was placed on service providers to develop community-based program alternatives and to reduce the number of individuals, particularly within the realms of mental health and developmental disabilities who were placed in institutional care (Taylor, 2001). Major legislation and policy initiatives also took place during that time that directly related to children with disabilities.

In 1974, Elementary and Secondary Education Amendments of 1974 (P.L. 93-380) included amendments to Part B of the Education of the Handicapped Act (EHA) that laid the basis for comprehensive planning, the delivery of additional financial assistance to the states, and the protection of handicapped children's rights. In 1974, The Community Services Act (P.L. 93-644) broadened the focus of the Head Start Program by stipulating that 10% of children enrolled must be children with disabilities (Haworth, State of Michigan, Department of Labor and Economic Growth Website, 2004).

In 1975, two major pieces of legislation were passed. The Equal Education for All Handicapped Children Act (P.L. 94-142) established the right to a free and appropriate public education for all children with disabilities, ages 3 through 21, in the least restrictive environment possible. First signed in 1975 and modified regularly throughout the 1980's and 1990's, this legislation is currently referred to as the Individuals with Disabilities Education Act (IDEA) (P.L.100-476) (U.S. Department of Health and Human Services, Administration for Children and Families, Index of Federal Child Welfare Laws, 2004). Also passed in 1975, The Developmental Disabilities Assistance and Bill of Rights Act (P.L. 94-103) created a "bill of rights" and funded services for persons with developmental disabilities (Haworth, State of Michigan, Department of Labor and Economic Growth Disability Policy Website, 2004).

During the 1970s, major legislative and policy reforms also took place within the realm of child welfare. In 1979, based on the strong, persistent efforts of Native American/American Indian advocates, the Indian Child Welfare Act (P.L. 95-608) was passed by Congress. This act established minimum federal standards for the removal of Indian children from their families (extended families) and directed efforts to examine the feasibility of providing Indian children with schools near their homes (Library of Congress, Thomas on the Internet, 2004). This legislation served as a major catalyst for the passage of The Adoption Assistance and Child Welfare Act of 1980 (P.L. 96-272). This law authorized appropriations for adoption and foster care assistance to the states and required states to provide adoption assistance "to parents who adopt a child who is AFDC-eligible and is a child with special needs" (U.S. Department of Health and Human Services, 2004). Also, in 1980, The Civil Rights of Institutionalized Persons Act (P.L. 96-247) authorized the U. S. Department of Justice to sue states for alleged violations of the rights of institutionalized persons, including persons in mental hospitals or facilities for people with mental retardation (Haworth, State of Michigan, Department of Labor and Economic Growth Disability Policy Website, 2004).

Emergence of the Family-Centered Approach

In 1986, The Education of the Handicapped Act Amendments (P.L. 99-457) included a new grant program for states to develop an early intervention system specifically for infants and toddlers with disabilities and their families and provide greater incentives for states to provide preschool programs for children with disabilities between the ages of three and five (Dunst, 2002).

In June of 1997, amendments were made to the IDEA (P.L.105-17) and in March of 1999, the final Department of Education Regulations was issued (Altshuler & Kopels, 2003). Part C of these amendments, pertaining to the early intervention system, expanded the role of parents in the educational system and promoted a family-centered approach to service provision for children with disabilities. Family centered early intervention philosophy and strategies draw from a strengths based perspective which encourages partnerships, family choice, and the provision of the support and information necessary for parents to become advocates for the child and family (Bruder, 2000). Family centered practice is flexible, individualized, collaborative, and acknowledges the longevity of the family's involvement with the child (Mahoney, Boyce, Fewell, Spiker & Wheeden, 1999) with the goal of providing services and support to families in order for them to support their child's development and maintain family functioning (Dunst, 2002). A family-centered model not only values the participation of the family in the development of the individualized family service plan (IFSP), but also supports family partnerships in program and policy development in the early intervention system and in other educational settings as well (Dunst, 2002).

During the 1990s, through the use of "mainstreaming" and inclusion models as well as community residence and independent and assisted living programs, continued efforts have been undertaken to more effectively integrate children and adolescents with disabilities into educational systems (Heubert, Harvard Education Letter, 1994). In 1999, further revisions made in the IDEA strengthened the role of families in the educational process providing more opportunities for participation by mandating that the Individualized Education Plan (IEP) included information regarding additional strategies used to involve the parent beyond IEP meetings (U.S. Department of Education, 2004). The IEP concept also relates well to "person-centered" planning which also emerged during the 1990s and places a much stronger emphasis on the interrelationship between the individual with a disability and the environment, including caregivers and service providers as well as increasing consumer involvement in all aspects of service planning and delivery (Onken, 1997).

The 1999 revisions of the IDEA expanded the social workers' role in a school setting, while maintaining states' rights to establish their own standards for service provision such as whether or not social work services to children and families with disabilities will be provided by the schools or not. The term "social work services in schools" now includes but is not limited to: preparing a social or developmental history on a child with a disability, group and/or individual counseling with the child and family, and working in partnership with parents and others on those aspects of a child's living situation (school, home, community) that affect the child's adjustment in school (Altshuler & Kopels, 2003, p. 327).

Despite these changes, studies have indicated that attending and participating in IEP meetings at the local school level is often an unpleasant experience for parents, especially when they perceive a lack of receptivity to their input and ideas. Altshuler and Kopels (2003) indicate that social workers, as knowledgeable advocates for parents, are in a better position to ensure that parent's voices are heard during such meetings. In addition to this, depending on the scope of the school social worker's functions as defined by a particular school district, s/he can also further assist parents by assuming a "case coordinator/manager" role and tracking the actual involvement of the broad range of school staff that may be involved in implementing the IEP, "trouble shooting" issues pertaining to inconsistent or lack of follow-through, and advocating for required enforcement of the IDEA with the Chairs of and Committee on Special Education.

Though understanding how the family-centered approach is utilized in educational settings is of importance, it is also important to consider the extent of utilization of this approach in other settings. For example, the nursing profession supported the concept of family-centered care even before its advent in early intervention (Darbyshire, 1993). Families of children with disabilities are often involved with the medical system relating to matters of diagnosis, acute care, critical care related to chronic medical conditions, routine care, and various therapeutic services. However, the first major point of contact for some families is that of the Neonatal Intensive Care Unit (NICU). Though all infants who spend time in the NICU do not have developmental disabilities, the NICU experience is often the beginning of the medical parent/professional relationship for many families who have children born with congenital disabilities.

Such units are highly specialized, technology driven, critical care environments where the importance of family involvement is essential. Since, however, the medical model traditionally focuses on the individual patient it has not necessarily supported the family in its role as collaborative partner and informed decision maker, both components of family-centered practice. In such environments, physicians may expect to make the decisions while nurses and therapists are expected to carry out the treatment. However, those family members not seen as "visitors" are expected to respond in much the same way as professionals by assuming care giving and care management roles (keeping charts, feeding, positioning, etc.). If family members attempt to take a break, they may be labeled as not caring or as abandoning not only the child, but also the staff who have grown to rely on them for respite and to supplement the provision of direct care to their child due to under-staffing or staffing shortages.

Some strides do, however, appear to have been made. For example, in a study of 11 medical center NIC Units whose staff collaborated in a family-centered care project, centers began to shift from seeing parents as visitors to parents as partners in their child's care. The units developed family-centered philosophy of care statements and developed or expanded family advisory councils (Cisneros Moore, Coker, DuBuisson, Swett & Edwards, 2003). Knight has also found that the concept of "family-centered nursing care" has been adopted in some medical settings and supports the philosophy that the family is a central figure in the care of the child (Knight, 1995, Newton, 2000).

Family-centered practice is purported to guide social work in child welfare and mental health systems. The creation of the Child and Adolescent Service System Program (CASSP) in the mental health system in 1984 was an initiative that emphasized the involvement of families in all mental health planning and service delivery (Stroul & Friedman, 1994). This initiative represented a shift in thinking away from placing the blame on parents for the child's problem. However, a national study conducted by Johnson et al. (2003) indicated that 40% of social workers reported that they felt that parents were responsible for their child's social/behavioral disability. In addition, they felt that gathering information from families was important to give workers an idea about family systems and dynamics, but not as part of a collaborative or partnership endeavor. Thus, while family dynamics were seen as contributing to the social and emotional difficulties of the child, soliciting greater family involvement as an intervention tool was not seen as viable in working with the family.

Bailey, Buysse, Edmondson and Smith (1992) also identify family choice and family priorities as inherent in a family-centered philosophy. Though family choice may not always be totally attainable in some service settings, being sensitive to family desires without trying to change or force them to match the prescribed roles and functions of the service system is an important role of the social worker. Social workers in these settings need to assume a stronger role in actively promoting the integration of a family-centered approach through familiarizing themselves with the major risk and protective factors associated with the experiences of such families as well as the particular cultures of the environments that families with children or adolescents with disabilities co-exist, function within, and participate in.

In addition to possible biases that social work practitioners in the field might hold towards the use of a family-centered approach, another factor that may hinder greater utilization of this approach is the lack of access that new social work practitioners entering the field have, via some of the more current social work human behavior and generalist practice texts, to content on family-centered practice. For example, while a targeted review of texts indicated that disability content, overall, is represented in varying degrees in these texts, only minor content was found on the individual child or adolescent within the broader context of the family, on the experiences of such families as a unit, or on the family-centered approach (Hutchison, 2003, Zastrow, 2004).

In addition to providing a fair amount of content on disability that is interspersed throughout the text, Schriver (2004) does present content that relates directly to families of children and adolescents with disabilities. Such content is predominantly from the vantage point of developmental assessment tools that can be applied to identification of disabilities/ disabling conditions as well as a brief overview of research on culturally diverse families (Harry, 2002) that has been generalized to families and disability and issues related to service delivery. However, other than a reference to the link between "family-centered practice" and early intervention and a brief overview of "challenges" facing families, no further content on this approach is presented. Mackelprang and Salsgiver (1999) focus exclusively on disability. References to the families of individuals with disabilities are interspersed throughout the text, including the integration of content on family perspectives into the chapter on life stage development. However, the chapter on assessment and human service practice does not include any reference to or content on utilization of the "family-centered" approach; nor are any references to this approach included in any other section.

A Family-Centered Framework

While integrating a family-centered approach into social work practice with families of children and adolescents with disabilities does not yet appear to have been fully embraced, its congruence with the principles of strengths-based social work practice which emphasizes client strengths and resources as well as developing a collaborative client-worker relationship (Saleeby, 1992) makes it an appropriate construct to utilize in working with families of children and adolescents with disabilities and one that warrants further development. One of the difficulties that must begin to be more effectively addressed is the need for a conceptual framework that provides a succinct, yet comprehensive overview of the major aspects of the range of possible experiences of families of children and adolescents with disabilities needs to be considered, understood, and integrated into current frameworks for approaching data collection, assessment, and intervention. Table 1: *A Family-Centered Framework for Exploring the Experiences of Families of Children and Adolescents with Disabilities* provides a comprehensive, although certainly not exhaustive overview, of the major components of a conceptual construct that may be utilized for integrating the actual application of a family-centered approach into social work practice with children and adolescents with disabilities and their families. This framework will also, hopefully, set the stage for further exploration, research, development, implementation and evaluation of ways in which the family-centered approach as it relates such families can be more effectively integrated into social work practice efforts.

Table 1 is broken down into three major segments: the family as a unit and parents as primary caregivers, the child/adolescent, and the sibling/s. Some of the major factors that warrant exploration are identified in each segment. It should be noted that, rather than being utilized as a diagnostic or prescriptive tool, this framework is meant to be *a starting point* from which to more fully assess *from the vantage point of the child, parent/s, and sibling/s (individually and collectively)* the actual relevance/significance of that aspect from each of their own perspectives. In addition to this, while, at first glance, some aspects noted appear to be repetitive across the three segments of the table, in actuality, each aspect must also be explored within the context of the unique experiences of each family member.

While providing an explanation of each aspect of this framework lies beyond the scope of this chapter, further explanation is needed of some of the major underlying constructs that might serve as guiding principles for its implementation. In addition to this, some of the research findings that pertain to each of the major components (the family unit and parent as primary caregivers, the child, and sibling/s) that provide a context in which to "ground" the aspects outlined pertaining to each component follows.

While the majority of the terms outlined in Table 1 are self-explanatory, the terms "congenital" and "acquired" disability warrant further explanation. Congenital disabilities may best be understood from the vantage point of risk factors. Berger (1994) (as cited in Shriver, 2004) identifies

TABLE 1. A Framework for Exploring the Experiences of Families of Children and Adolescents with Disabilities

Factors Related to Family Unit/Parents As Primary Caregivers	Factors Related To Individual Child/ Adolescent	Factors Related to Sibling/s
• Nature of parent/s relationship with partner • Extent of relationship/marital harmony prior to birth of child/onset of disability • SES/social class • Previous risk factors unrelated to any disability-specific stressors • Perceived roles related to gender/age of adults and children • Life stage/s of family as a unit • Nature of relationships within family as a unit and among individual family members • Family decision making patterns • Family communication patterns • Extent and nature of involvement with any other child/ren prior to birth of child/onset of disability • Preconceived notions on disability (general/disability-specific) • Knowledge and understanding of child's disability & implications • Extent of feelings of grief & loss/Initial adjustment to disability • Long-term adjustment/extent of co-existing grief & loss • Parents' sense of efficacy • Extent of synchronicity/acceptance of one another's feelings, views, coping strategies • Ability to spend time and provide support to sibling/s • Perspectives on disability based on race, ethnicity, culture	• Age • Individual life stage at time of assessment • Birth order • Nature of relationship with parents as a unit and each individual parent • Nature of relationship with each sibling • Gender and gender role expectations • Nature (congenital/acquired) and type of disability • Visible, Non-visible, Hidden Disability • Individual life stage at onset of disability (congenital/acquired) • History of developmental functioning/ assessment of developmental assets (physical/cognitive/social/emotional) • Self concept/sense of identity (strengths/ abilities) prior to onset of disability (if acquired) • Extent of peer involvement and nature of social/emotional support from peers • Perceived stress/concerns • Feelings of grief/loss (based on age of onset and circumstances surrounding disability/as individual progresses through childhood and adolescence) • Current self-concept/sense of identity • Current feelings related to self-esteem • Life expectations/life goals (as able to be expressed by each child/adolescent)	• Age • Birth Order • Gender and Gender role expectations • Individual life stage • History of Developmental Functioning/ Assessment of developmental assets (physical/cognitive/social/ emotional/ spiritual) • Nature of relationships with parent/s and any other sibling/s prior to birth of child/onset of disability • Feelings of grief/loss (initial) • Knowledge and understanding of sibling's disability and implications (long-term grief and loss) • Expectations of sibling who is disabled • Perceived stress/concerns related to sibling with disability • Perceived stress/concerns related to current relationship with parent/s (after onset) • Current nature of individual relationships with any other sibling/s • Peer relationships including perceptions of sibling who is disabled, extent of social acceptance, and nature and availability of on-going support • Perceptions/level of interaction of significant other (dating/partner)

• Religious/spiritual perspectives on disability • Access to affordable, accessible housing and physical environment • Extent of health care resources, overall, and related to specific disability of child/adolescent • Availability and use of social/emotional support including extended family, fictive kinship • Extent of availability & access to transportation, respite services • Beliefs about seeking/receiving help • Extent of involvement with outside systems (education, health care, child welfare, developmental disabilities) • Overall strengths/Areas of resiliency of family/parents	• Coping strategies (specific to context of disability, general) • Current knowledge and understanding of disability and possible implications • Quality and nature of involvement with educational system • Quality and nature of involvement with other outside systems • Overall strengths of child/Areas of resiliency	• Extent of interaction between sibling who is disabled and other sibling/s within educational, social, recreational and other systems • Current knowledge and understanding of disability and possible implications • Coping strategies (general/specific to context of specific disability) • Overall strengths of sibling/Areas of resiliency

NOTE: Though some factors are similar across family members, it is important to understand the unique response of each individual in relation to each area in order to understand the family response as a unit. Support and intervention must be led by the family based on their identified needs, strengths and priorities.

established risks as "conditions that include neurological, genetic ortho-pedic, cognitive, or sensory impairments or other physical or medical syndromes" (p. 174). Such conditions may be linked to genetic predis-positions and/or to the prenatal period of fetal development. Berger (1994) (as cited in Schriver, 2004) identifies biological risks as "conditions that are physical or medical trauma experiences that occur in the prenatal pe-riod, during the birth process, or in the neonatal period" (p. 174). Such conditions may be correctable, result in developmental delays, or mani-fest as permanent disabilities in later life stages as the child continues to grow and develop. While in some instances, acquired disabilities may overlap with conditions defined as "biological risks," such disabilities can occur at any point during an individuals' life course.

The framework also references the terms "visible," "non-visible," and "hidden" disabilities. While the term "visible" disability, at first glance, may appear to be self-explanatory, the underlying dynamics related to the distinctions between each of these constructs is actually very com-plex and an in-depth explanation would extend beyond the scope of this chapter. However, one major distinction that is important to articulate is that with "visible" disabilities, the focus is more on what DePoy and French Gilson (2004) refer to as "legitimacy from without" based on how others define disability and/or may treat others who do not fit dis-ability designations while "non-visible disabilities" relate more to the construct of "legitimacy from within." From this vantage point, the focus is on how the individual who has been defined by others as disabled de-fines disability legitimacy and response from her/his own vantage point. (For more background on Explanatory Legitimacy Theory, see section on "Siblings" later in this article.)

In contrast, the concept of "hidden disabilities" relates more to the in-ternal process that an individual who is defined as disabled by others may experience with regard to internalizing a positive sense of disabil-ity identity through engaging in a series of processes as they integrate disability into one's self image. Onken and Mackelprang (1997) (as cited by Mackelprang and Salsgiver, 1999) draw from the literature pertain-ing to sexual minorities and the "coming out" process and outline six processes, that while not stages or sequential in nature, may be applied to the experiences of persons who may be struggling and/or seeking to integrate disability into an overall sense of identity: (1) Pre-awareness conformity; (2) Denial or avoidance; (3) Comparison; (4) Confusion and dissonance; (5) Immersion and resistance; (6) Acceptance and Pride; and (7) Introspection and synthesis (for more background on these processes, see *Disability: A Diversity Model in Human Service Practice, 1999*).

It should be noted that the concept of "hidden disabilities" relate to an internal struggle that may only take place with individuals who feel a need to rectify discrepancies in experiences that relate to what DePoy and French Gilson (2004) have conceptualized as "legitimacy from without" and "legitimacy from within."

Whether from an Explanatory Legitimacy Theory perspective (French Gilson, 2004), Identity Formation Theory perspective (Mackelprang & Onken, 1997), life stage or developmental perspective, it is important for the social worker who is engaging in the use of a family-centered approach to explore with the child/adolescent who is disabled as well as other members of the family unit perceptions of disability as a developmental, social, environmental, and political construct and the implications that this may have with regard to need identification, goals, and resources.

INDIVIDUAL CHILD:
SOME ADDITIONAL CONSIDERATIONS

While the emphasis of this chapter is on integrating a family-centered approach into working with families of children and adolescents with disabilities, any such approach must, of course, also incorporate a "person-centered" focus (Onken, 1997) and start with the individual child or adolescent. Shonkuff, Hauser-Cram, Kraus, and Upshur (1992) (as cited in Kirby & Fraser, 2000) indicate that longitudinal research on the development of young children with disabilities is sparse. Given this, a growing body of research that may be useful to draw from is that of risk and resilience. Kirby and Fraser (2000) provide an overview of some of the major differences in risk and protective factors among children with disabilities. A study by Knitzer and Aber (1995) (as cited in Kirby & Fraser, 2000) indicated that there is general agreement that children living in poverty are at significant risk of various developmental difficulties. Type of disability and age were also identified as major risk factors.

A study done by Werner with colleagues in Kauai (1990) (as cited in Kirby & Fraser, 2000) indicated that factors that might promote resilience in children with disabilities may vary by gender, with resilient girls seeming to come from households that provided consistent support and emphasized risk taking and independence while resilient boys came from households in which emotional expressiveness was encouraged, greater structure and supervision were provided, and a male role model.

Another construct that may be useful to draw from when focusing on the possible needs of the child is that of developmental assets. Through extensive research, Search Institute (2004) has identified 40 building blocks of healthy development that help young people grow up healthy, caring and responsible. These building blocks are divided into two major categories: External Assets and Internal Assets. In addition to outlining external assets that relate to the family, peers, the school, and the community, commitment to learning, positive values, social competence and positive identity are highlighted as major areas of internal assets/essential building blocks. Search Institute has blended the literature on child development and this framework of assets that was originally focused on adolescents to identify parallel, developmentally appropriate sets of assets for infants, toddlers, preschoolers, and elementary age children. While this material does not focus specifically on children and adolescents with disabilities, it does provide a strengths-based, person-in-environment, family and child-centered framework that might be tailored to the specific experiences of children with disabilities and their families.

Positive identity does appear to be an aspect of development that has been explored to some extent in relation to children and adolescents with disabilities. In recent studies of self-esteem of children and adolescents with disabilities Antle (2004) found that participants reported self worth at similar levels as found in their peers without disabilities. Strong parent support was identified as a strong protective factor for the young adult even though it may contradict traditional thinking about the "launching stage" (Germain, 1994). Self worth was also related to perceived support from close friends. Children and adolescents with disabilities may need assistance in developing social skills, overcoming physical barriers related to relationship building (such as transportation to friend's homes (Antles, 2004)) as well as coping with the isolation that sometimes occurs when peers are uncomfortable with the differences.

DePoy and French Gilson (2004) discuss the interrelationship between Explanatory Legitimacy Theory and disability cultural identity. The action element of legitimacy for individuals involves both a sense of identity and cultural belonging and influenced by factors such as responses to self and responses to others. From this vantage point, positive identity formation for the child or adolescent with a disability may be fostered both by the ways in which peers are responding to the disability as well as by how the adolescent with the disability is conceptualizing their own sense of identity and experiences that either contribute to or hinder (such as marginalization, oppression, discrimination) a broader sense of cultural belonging.

The Family Unit and Parents as Main Caregivers: Some Major Considerations

When considering the needs of families of children and adolescents with disabilities, additional factors need to be explored with regard to the overall functioning of the family as a unit. In a study conducted by Smith, Oliver, and Innocenti (2001), it was found that programs and services need to focus on facilitating parent's identification of their own as well as the broader family's specific needs and resources. Such an approach provides families with the foundation on which strategies needed to cope with the on-going demands of raising a child with a major disability can be built.

Recent literature cites that families of children with disabilities do experience more stress than children without disabilities (Dyson, 1998, Hadadian, 1994). This seems to be consistent across the literature that pertains to a range of conditions including physical and intellectual disabilities (Boyce, Behl, Mortensen & Akers, 1991; Innocenti, Huh & Boyce, 1992), visual impairment (Troster, 2001), and traumatic brain injury (Ergh, Rapport, Coleman & Hanks, 2001).

Though a variety of factors have been identified as contributing to overall family stress such as severity of disability (Smith et al., 2001) financial resources (Innocenti et al., 1992, Mahoney, O'Sullivan & Robinson, 1992), and prior family functioning (Smith et al., 2001), behavioral and care demands of the child seem to be particularly related to caregiver stress (Innocenti et al., 1992; Britner, Morog, Pianta & Marvin, 2003; Keller & Honig, 2004; Smith et al., 2001). Though placement in a residential setting was once the primary option for families of children with moderate or severe disabilities, this trend has been changing since the early 1970s. Most of the time, the young child lives at home and will be cared for by the family. This requires a shift in orientation for the family as well as for the medical, educational and social service community. Complex, time-consuming regimes of care or treatment may be necessary in order to reduce complications and enhance the child's quality of life. Strong emphasis continues to be placed on family-based care and supplemental care support models that rely heavily on the immediate family to serve as the primary care giver, case manager, advocate and service provider.

While stress may be very specific to the nature of the child's disability and the overall demands placed on the family, grief, as a major dynamic, is reported to be one of the aspects of the parent's life experiences that may distinguish them from other parents. In the past, programs have focused on specific parent reactions related to grief stages (Garguilo, 1985) with the goal of final adjustment. Seligman and Darling (1989) however, reported that symptoms of grief may occur throughout the family life cycle. This notion of coexisting grief and acceptance was supported in a study of aging mothers of adult children with disabilities (Keller, 2004). The mothers reported that accepting the reality of the disability and the sadness that it sometimes triggers was an important step in adaptation and coping. Though shock and sadness are documented consistently as part of the initial reaction to a child's disability, and can occur throughout the life cycle, coping and adaptation and even positive transformation (Scorgie & Sobsey, 2000) is reported by many families.

Family life stage is a significant factor for social workers to explore when assessing the needs of families of children and adolescents with disabilities. Four stages in the family life cycle have been identified by Turnbull and Turnbull (1990). These include early childhood (birth through five years), school age (six through 12 years), adolescence (13 through 21 years), and adulthood (21 years and older). Adaptation to a child's disability is a life long process that occurs within the context of the family's developmental cycle. Transitions and unanticipated events that occur during the typical family developmental life cycle may cause increased stress for families of children with disabilities. Though change over time is an obvious developmental concept, for many families having a child with a congenital disability poses a unique set of stressors and strains including cumulative stress and caregiver fatigue and burnout. For families of children with acquired disabilities, depending on the circumstances, the major disruption and trauma that has occurred within the context of the family's developmental life cycle related to the onset of the disability often results in major changes within the family and has long-term effects on the entire family system as well as each individual family member.

Grant, Nolan and Keady (2003) present a model of thinking that focuses on family constructs representing events/activity related to the family response of a child or adolescent with a disability rather on developmental stages. Constructs include: (1) Building on the past; (2) Recognizing the need; (3) Taking it on; (4) Working through it; (5) Reaching the end; and (6) A new beginning provide an applicable framework to support families irregardless of age of onset of disability.

Both the family life stages and developmental models identify the need for social workers to be aware of the interactive quality on the child's developmental state, the family life cycle and the family response in order to support parents and family as a unit through the transitions and changes that will occur in their lives.

Demographic characteristics of the family such as ethnicity, culture, SES and social class has also been found to effect family response including coping ability and meaning that is attributed to having a child with a disability (Dunst, Trivette & Cross, 1986; Houser & Seligman, 1991). The importance of ethnicity and culture as it relates to adaptation of families to disabilities has been recently identified (Hanline & Daley, 1992; Huer, Saez & Doan, 2001; Parette, Huer & Wyatt, 2001). Cultural beliefs can effect the coping strategies of a family in response to a disability (Rogers, Dulan & Blacher, 1995) as well as determining short and long-term goals.

Harry (2002) links the emphasis on issues of culturally diverse families of children with disabilities to the advent of family centered practice in early intervention supported by PL 99-457 in 1986. Prior to this time, family roles were conceptualized in ways congruent with white, middle class families, i.e., psychoanalytical model (grief and sorrow) and later the parent as the teacher approach, a family-allied model (Carey, Lewis, Farris & Burns, 1998; Epstein & Lee, 1995). Since the child's disability provided the identification for minority status, culture, language or any other unique status of the family was ignored.

Stronger emphasis has been placed on examining the experiences of culturally diverse families of children and adolescents with disabilities. In a study comparing Asian American family perceptions with European American families Asians attribute etiology of disability to supernatural sources or ancestral sins with resulting feelings of guilt, shame and need to protect child (Parette, Chang & Huer, 2004). In addition, Asian American families demonstrate a high regard for the educational system including a reluctance to take on decision making roles (Chan, 1997). There does seem to be variations within broad cultural groups. In a study of families of young children with communication disabilities, Parett, Chauag and Huer (2004) found that Chinese families may have different views that those of other Asian families. The Chinese families reported general acceptance of the child's disability, they viewed educational programs as being important but also were able to express dissatisfaction with services. These families actively participated in decision-making at meetings and were well informed of legal rights.

Though it is important for practitioners to understand specific beliefs related to family values, child development, coping strategies as well as the meaning of disability of a particular group, care must by taken not to generalize an individual family's response to the culture group and promote culture stereotypes (Ow, Tan & Goh, 2004; Rogers, Dulan & Blacher, 1995). Harry (2002) argues for a contextual understanding of cultural diversity, being aware of broad cultural implications related to disability but also understanding the individual family's beliefs, values and concerns. In addition, it is important for the social worker to understand that the basis of their professional beliefs about disability and family response to disability may be cultural (Harry, 2002) or systemic, but not necessarily universal.

Siblings

Inherent in a discussion of families of children and adolescents with a disability are siblings. Children learn many social skills from their siblings, their first social network. Sibling relationships are the basis of interactions with people outside the family and tend to be characterized by supportiveness, concern and mutual affection. Family-centered practice should emphasize the importance of considering how the sibling/s may be influenced by life experiences that relate specifically to having a sibling with a disability. The strengths, stressors and areas of resiliency demonstrated by the sibling/s should also be explored when discussing family goals and strategies.

While some research has been conducted on siblings, one of the difficulties inherent in the current research is that it sometimes produces findings that are contradictory or hard to generalize, due to the fact that it is usually very disability-specific (developmental, intellectual, etc.) While further study is needed, an examination of some of the current findings that appear to "cut across" the different experiences of siblings include feelings of loneliness and grief (Wolf, Fisman, Ellison & Freeman, 1998; Opperman & Alant, 2003), feelings of guilt and shame (Opperman & Alant, 2003) and not having enough information about the child's disability or its implications for the family (Opperman & Alant, 2003; Williams et al., 2002). However, Rivers and Stoneman (2003) also found that siblings without disabilities can develop positive relationships with their siblings with disabilities. Positive outcomes reported include acceptance of differences in others and pro-social interactions (Benson, Gross & Kellum, 1999; Dyson, 1998). Research conducted by Pitten Cate and Loots (2000) also indicated that other positive experiences reported by siblings had to do with the development of their own insight including acquiring a different perspective towards people, especially people with disabilities.

Though the impact on the sibling can also be influenced by the type of disability, birth order, age, life stage of sibling when child acquired disability, and gender of the sibling, the major factors that seem to influence positive outcomes are family functioning, adaptation, family communication and coping styles (Benson et al., 1999; Fisman, Wolf, Ellison & Freeman, 2000; Williams et al., 2002). Cate and Loots (2000) also reference several studies that suggest that parents demonstrated acceptance of the child with a disability as well as conveyed positive attitudes are often adopted by siblings, and are therefore of importance to sibling interactions. Sibling support groups (Dyson, 1998; McLinden, 1990) may also provide necessary information and peer support for school age siblings.

CONCLUSION

Originating from the early intervention system, the use of a family-centered approach to service provision for young children with disabilities has been expanded, in educational as well as pediatric medicine, child welfare and child mental health settings, to include middle school age children and adolescents and their families. While this approach is being utilized by some social work practitioners, in general, social work has been slow to embrace the utilization of family-centered practice within the context of working with families of children and adolescents with disabilities. A major factor that may play a role in influencing greater utilization of this approach is the need to better integrate, into social work data collection, assessment and intervention, a conceptual framework that social workers can use as a tool for guiding the exploration of the range of possible factors that may have a role in shaping the experiences, needs and goals of these families as well as intervention strategies. Drawing from the framework provided, social workers need to:

- Acknowledge and actively promote parents as primary partners in the care of their child
- Provide the information, skills training and resources needed to support full family participation
- Develop collaborative working relationships that actively engage the child, parent/s and family unit as equal partners

- Utilize, within the context of a family-centered approach, a person-centered planning model for addressing the needs of the child/adolescent with a disability
- Acknowledge and assess the needs of sibling/s including what actual resources and supports must be provided to assist families in effectively addressing such needs.
- Support the right of families to make choices, set priorities, and identify the resources needed to enhance the functioning of the overall family as a unit
- Provide information and skills so that families can make informed decisions and assume the amount of responsibility that is best for them
- Empower families to become advocates or work as an advocate for the family
- Work as an interdisciplinary member of the team that includes family members are viable, fully participating members
- Infuse, into a family-centered approach, cultural competence by continually drawing from emerging research and other knowledge bases that focus on common themes that may be "woven across the life fabric" of diverse families of children/adolescents with disabilities while striving to ensure that the individuality and uniqueness of each family's experience is still retained.

REFERENCES

Allard, M. A., Howard, M. A., Vorderer, L. E., & Wells, A. I. (Eds.). (1999). *Ahead of his time: Selected speeches of Gunnar Dybwad.* Washington, DC: American Association on Mental Retardation.

Altshuler, S., & Kopels, S. (1993). Advocating in schools for children with disabilities: What's new with IDEA? *Social Work, 48*(3), 320-329.

Antle, B. (2004). Factors associated with self-worth in young people with physical disabilities. *Health and Social Work, 29*(3), 167-175.

Bailey, D. B., Buysse, V., Edmondson, R., & Smith, T. M. (1992). Creating family-centered services in early intervention: Perceptions of professionals in four states. *Exceptional Children, 58,* 298-309.

Benson, B. A., Gross, A. M., & Kellum, G. (1999). The siblings of children with craniofacial anomalies. *Children's Health Care, 28*(1), 51-68.

Boyce, G. C., Behl, D., Mortensen, L., & Akers, J. (1991). Child characteristics, family demographics and family processes: Their effects on the stress experienced by families of children with disabilities. *Counseling Psychology Quarterly, 4,* 273-288.

Britner, P. A., Morog, M. C., Pianta, R. C., & Marvin, R. S. (2003). Stress and coping: A comparison of self-report measures of functioning in families of young children with cerebral palsy or no medical diagnosis. *The Journal of Child and Family Studies,* *12*(3), 335-348.

Bruder, M. B. (2000). Family-centered early intervention: Clarifying our values for the new millennium. *Topics in Early Childhood Special Education, 20*(2), 105-115.

Carey, N., Lewis, L., Farris, E., & Burns, S. (1998). *Parent involvment in children's education: Efforts by public elementary schools* (Report N. NCES 98-032). Washington, DC: U.S. Department of Education, Office of Educational Research and Improvement.

Cate, I. M. P., & Loots, G. M. P. (2000). Experiences of siblings of children with physical disabilities: An empirical investigation. *Disability & Rehabilitation., 22*(9), 399-408.

Cisneros Moore, K. A., Coker, K., DuBuisson, A. B., Swett, B., & Edwards, W. H. (2003). Implementing potentially better practices for improving family-centered care in neonatal intensive care units: Successes and Challenges. *Pediatrics, 111*(4) 450-460.

Darbyshire, R. (1993) Parents, nurses and pediatric nursing: A critical review. *Journal of Advanced Nursing, 18*, 1670-1680.

Department of Labor and Economic Growth, *Events in the Development of Disability Policy* retrieved 1/10/05 *from* http://www.michigan.gov/mdcd/0,1607,7-122-25392_25407_31089-12437—,00.html

DePoy, E. & French Gilson, S. (2004). *Rethinking disability: Principles for professional and social change.* Monterey, California: Brooks/Cole Publishing Co.

Dunst, C. J. (2002). Family-centered practices: Birth through high school. *The Journal of Special Education, 36*(3) 139-147.

Dunst, C. J., Trivette, C. M., & Cross, A. H. (1986). Mediating influences of social support: Personal, family, and child outcomes. *American Journal of Mental Deficiency, 90*, 403-417.

Dyson, L. L. (1998). A support program for siblings of children with disabilities: What siblings learn and what they like. *Psychology in the Schools, 35*(1), 199.

Epstein, J., & Lee, S. (1995). *National patterns of school and family connections.* In B. Ryan, G.Adams, T. Gullota, R. Weissberg, & R. Hampton (Eds.). *The family-school connection: Theory, research and practice,* (pp. 108-154). Thousand Oaks, CA: Sage.

Ergh, T. C., Rapport, L. J., Coleman, R. D., & Hanks, R. A. (2002). Predictors of caregiver and family functioning following traumatic brain injury: Social support moderates caregiver distress. *Journal of Head Trauma Rehabilitation, 17*(2), 155-174.

Fisman, S., Wolf, L., Ellison, D., & Freeman, T. (2000). A longitudinal study of siblings of children with chronic disabilities. *Canadian Journal of Psychiatry, 45*(4), 369-375.

Frasher, M. K. (2000). Promoting the development of young children with disabilities. In M. K. Fraser (Ed.) *Risk and resilience in childhood: An ecological perspective* (pp. 244-264). Washington, D.C.: NASW Press.

Garguilo, R. M. (1985). *Working with parents of exceptional children: A guide for professionals.* Boston: Houghton Mifflin.

Germain, C. B. (1994). Emerging conceptions of family development over the life course. *Families in Society, 75*, 259-267.

Grant, G., Molan, M., & Keady, J. (2003). Supporting families over the life course: Mapping temporality. *Journal of Intellectual Disability Research, 47*, 342-351.

Hadadian, A. (1994). Stress and social support in fathers and mothers of young children with and without disabilities. *Early Education and Development, 5,* 227-235.

Hanline, M. F., & Daley, S. E. (1992). Family coping strategies and strengths in Hispanic, African-American and Caucasian families of young children. *Topics in Early Childhood Special Education, 12*(3), 351-366.

Harry, B. (2002). Trends and issues in serving culturally diverse families of children with disabilities. *Journal of Special Education, 36*(3), 131-138.

Heubert, J. (1994). "Point/Counterpoint: Assumptions underlie arguments about inclusion." Harvard Education Letter, July/August, pg. 17.

Heur, M. B., Saenz, T., & Doan, J. H. D. (2001). Understanding the Vietnamese–American community: Implications for training educational personnel providing services to children with disabilities. *Communication Disorders Quarterly, 23,* 27-39.

Houser, R., & Seligman, M. (1991). A comparison of stress and coping by fathers of adolescents with mental retardation and fathers of adolescents without mental retardation. *Research in Developmental Disabilities, 12,* 251-260.

Hutchison, E. D. (2003). Dimensions of human behavior: The changing life course. Thousand Oaks, CA: Sage Publications.

Innocenti, M. S., Huh, K., & Boyce. G. C. (1992). Families of children with disabilities: Normative data and other considerations on parenting stress. *Topics in Early Childhood Special Education, 12,* 403-427.

Johnson, H. C., Cournoyer, D. E., Fliri, J., Flynn, M., Grant, A. M., Lant, M. A., Parasco, S., & Stanek, E. J. (2003). Are we parent-friendly? Views of parents of children with emotional and behavioral disabilities. *Families in Society, 84*(1), 95-108.

Keller, D. (2004, March). *Integrity vs. despair: Perceptions of mothers of adult children with disabilities.* Poster session presented at the annual meeting of the National Gerontological Social Work Conference, Anaheim, CA.

Keller, D., & Honig, A. S. (2004). Maternal and paternal stress in families with school-aged children with disabilities. *American Journal of Orthopsychiatry, 74*(3), 337-348.

Knight, L. (1995). Negotiating care roles. *Nursing Times, 91,* 31-33.

Mackelprang, R., & Salsgiver, R. (1999). *Disability: A diversity model approach in human service practice.* Pacific Grove, CA: Brooks/Cole.

Mahoney, G., Boyce, G., Fewell, R. R., Spiker, D., & Wheeden, C. A. (1998). The relationship of parent-child interaction to the effectivenss of early intervention services for at risk children with disabilities. *Topics in Early Childhood Special Education, 18,* 5-17.

Mahoney, G., O'Sullivan, P., & Robinson, C. (1992). The family environments of children with disabilities: Diverse but not so different. *Topics in Early Childhood Special Education, 12*(3), 386-402.

McLinden, S. E. (1990). Mothers' and fathers' reports of the effects of a young child with special needs on the family. *Journal of Early Intervention, 14,* 249-259.

Newton, M. S. (2000). Family-centered care: Current realities in parent participation. *Pediatric Nursing, 26*(2), 164-168.

Onken, S. (1997). Person-center planning in *Disability Resource Curriculum,* University of Texas. Presented at CSWE Annual Program Meeting, 1998.

Opperman, S., & Alant, E. (2003). The coping responses of the adolescent siblings of children with severe disabilities. *Disability & Rehabilitation, 35*(9), 441-454.

Ow, R., Tan, N. T., & Goh, S. (2004). Diverse perceptions of social support: Asian mothers of children with intellectual disability. *Families in Society: The Journal of Contemporary Social Services, 85*(2), 214-230.

Parrette, P., Chuang, S. L., & Huer, M. B. (2004). First-generation Chinese American families' attitudes regarding disabilities and educational interventions. *Focus on Autism and Other Developmental Disabilities,* 19(2), 114-123.

Parette, H. P., Huer, M. B., & Wyatt, T. A. (2002). Young African American children with disabilities and augmentative and alternative communication issues. *Early Childhood Education Journal, 29*(3), 201-207.

Rivers, J. W., & Stoneman, Z. (2003). Sibling relationships when a child has autism: Marital stress and support coping. *Journal of Autism and Developmental Disorders, 33*(4), 383-394.

Rogers-Dulan, J., & Blacher, J. (1995). African American families, religion and disability: A conceptual framework. *Mental Retardation, 33*(4), 226-238.

Saleeby, D. (Ed.). (1992). *The strengths perspective in social work practice.* New York: Longman.

Schriver, J. M. (2004). *Human behavior and the social environment: Shifting paradigms in essential knowledge for social work practice.* Boston: Allyn and Bacon.

Scorgie, K., & Sobsey, D. (2000). Transformational outcomes associated with parenting children who have disabilities. *Mental Retardation, 38*(3), 195-206.

Search Institute. Retrieved 1/10/05 from http//search-institute.org/assets/forty.html

Seligman, M., & Darling, R. B. (1989). *Ordinary families, special children: A systems approach to childhood disability.* New York: Guilford Press.

Smith, T. B., Oliver, M. N. I., & Innocenti, M. S. (2001). Parenting stress in families of children with disabilities. *American Journal of Orthopsychiatry, 71*(2), 257-261.

Stroul, B. A., & Friedman, R. M. (1994). *Introduction. Progress in children's mental health: A system of care for children and youth.* Washington, DC: Georgetown University Child Development Center, CASSP Technical Assistance Center.

Taylor, S. J. (2001). The continuum and current controversies in the USA. *Journal of Intellectual and Developmental Disability, 26*(1), 15-33.

Taylor, S. J., & Blatt, S. D. (Eds.). (1999). *In search of the promised land: The collected papers of Burton Blatt.* Washinton, DC: American Association on Mental Retardation.

Thomas on the Internet, retrieved 1/10/2005 from http://thomas.loc.gov/home/thomas.html

Troster, H. (2001). Sources of stress in mothers of young children with visual impairment. *Journal of Visual Impairment & Blindness, 95*(10), 623-637.

Turnbull, A. P., & Turnbull, H. R. (1990). Family life cycles. In A. P. Turnbull & H. R. Turnbull (Eds.), *Families, professionals and exceptionality: A special partnership.* New York: Merrill.

U. S. Department of Education. (n.d.) *History of the IDEA.* Retrieved November 17, 2004, from http://www.ed.gov/policy/speced/leg/idea/history.html

U. S. Department of Health and Human Services, Administration for Children and Families, Index of Federal Child Welfare Laws retrieved 1/10/05 from http://nccanch.acf.hhs.gov/general/legal/federal/federalchildlaws.cfm

Williams, P. D., Williams, A. R., Graff, J. C., Hanson, S., Staton, A., Hafeman, C. et al. (2002). Interrelationships among variables affecting well siblings and mothers in families of children with a chronic illness or disability. *Journal of Behavioral Medicine, 25*(5), 411-424.

Wolf, L. C., Fisman, S., Ellison, D., & Freeman, T. (1998). Effect of differential parental treatment in sibling dyads with one disabled child: A longitudinal perspective. *Journal of American Academy of Child and Adolescent Psychiatry, 37*, 1317-1325.

Zastrow, C. & Kirst-Ashman, K. (2004). *Understanding human behavior and the social environment.* Chicago: Nelson-Hall Publishers, Inc.

doi:10.1300/J198v06n01_07

Adjustment to Disability

Carol B. Cohen

Donna Napolitano

SUMMARY. This article will focus on the biopsychosocial challenges encountered when an individual is disabled at an early age as well as when an individual acquires a disability later in life. Two case examples will focus on the adaptations/life choices that are necessary to adequately meet psycho/social/developmental needs and enhance individual self esteem. The case of Rita, a woman who lost her hearing at age two, highlights the importance of integrating a biopsychosocial approach to understand the multiple challenges and adaptations of individuals who are disabled at an early age. Laureen, a woman who acquired a spinal cord injury during her late teen years, described her struggles as a young adult adapting to a physical disability. Both cases highlight the importance of integrating an ecological/systems framework focusing on a biopsychosocial perspective, emphasizing the interrelationship between biological, psychological, social, technological, cultural and political factors. doi:10.1300/J198v06n01_08 *[Article copies available for a fee from The Haworth Document Delivery Service: 1-800-HAWORTH. E-mail address: <docdelivery@haworthpress.com> Website: <http://www.HaworthPress.com> © 2007 by The Haworth Press, Inc. All rights reserved.]*

Carol B. Cohen, PhD, LCSW-C, is Associate Professor, Department of Social Work, Gallaudet University, 800 Florida Avenue NE, Washington, DC 20002 (E-mail: carol.cohen@gallaudet.edu). Donna Napolitano, c/o Gallaudet University, Department of Social Work, 800 Florida Avenue NE, Washington, DC 20002.

[Haworth co-indexing entry note]: "Adjustment to Disability." Cohen, Carol B., and Donna Napolitano. Co-published simultaneously in *Journal of Social Work in Disability & Rehabilitation* (The Haworth Press, Inc.) Vol. 6, No. 1/2, 2007, pp. 135-155; and: *Disability and Social Work Education: Practice and Policy Issues* (ed: Francis K. O. Yuen, Carol B. Cohen, and Kristine Tower) The Haworth Press, Inc., 2007, pp. 135-155. Single or multiple copies of this article are available for a fee from The Haworth Document Delivery Service [1-800-HAWORTH, 9:00 a.m. - 5:00 p.m. (EST). E-mail address: docdelivery@haworthpress.com].

KEYWORDS. Spinal cord injury, deafness, biopsychosocial framework, self esteem

ISSUES RELATED TO DEAFNESS

Approximately 90% of all deaf children are born to hearing parents (Schlesinger, 1978; Harvey, 1989). Those individuals who do not have any residual hearing will probably only be able to lip-read approximately 30% of all spoken language. Parents of young children may be doubly traumatized, not only by the diagnosis of deafness but by the many choices and contradictory advice related to surgical procedures, communication modalities as well as educational opportunities (Marschark, 1993, Harvey, 1989).

The primary caretaker usually assumes responsibility for meeting the basic needs of their infant which includes an opportunity to experience and begin to develop an internally derived sense of self. "The mother brings the world to the child" (St. Claire, 1996, p. 192). From a social constructivist framework, the attitude of parents (influenced by the stigma placed on disability) may greatly affect the parent-infant relationship. In addition, "studies of individual life courses, or the unfolding individual life experience over time, often focus on specific phases, reflecting how life courses are to a large extent culturally structured" (Sandvin, 2003, p. 6).

Hearing parents do not have the typical ways of engaging their deaf children. Communication challenges require parents to make major decisions related styles of communication and language development. The oral perspective focuses on an ability to speak and communicate orally. Assistive devices such as hearing aids, auditory loops or surgical procedures such as the cochlear implant facilitate the oral perspective. Another style focuses on visual communication, the use of American Sign Language (ASL) as the first language. Those who embrace ASL do not value the use of spoken language as a major component of the communication process. In addition, there are many variations of these perspectives including those who advocate for a bicultural/bilingual approach that focuses on both visual and auditory communication. The importance of language and communication is essential for ego and identity development. Glickman notes:

Without a solid language system the child lacks the major tools for relatedness with others and embeddedness in one's familial social context. The child also lacks major tools needed to think about himself or herself abstractly and therefore form an identity. (1996, p. 134)

The meaning of the disability may greatly affect the family's reaction to the child and thus have a great impact on the parenting process (attachment between infant and caregiver) that includes the choice of communication styles. Parents may grieve or mourn the loss of a child who is not "perfect" (Solomon, Springer, and Vachon, 1993). Some parents, in fact, deny the disability.

Rita is a 50-year-old deaf woman who cannot lip-read and who does not have an intelligible voice. Rita's hearing loss was acute. At the age of two, Rita was hospitalized due an infection that caused a high fever and lost her hearing overnight. Doctor's suspected that the antibiotics that were given to Rita contributed to the hearing loss. Rita's hearing loss was profound and she did not have any residual hearing, thus she could not lip-read.

Rita's parents made choices that did not meet the functional ability of their child. They were greatly influenced by the social/cultural influences of that time period which supported the basic tenets of "integration." Integration focused on an oral approach to deafness; an approach to minimize and hide differences in order to fit into the hearing able-bodied world. At the time technological advances that facilitate and enhance oral communication did not exist (such as the cochlear implant) and sign language was not a socially accepted language and embraced much stigmatism in the hearing world.

A sense of attachment is necessary in order to develop social competence, self esteem and resilience against stress/challenges (Huebner & Thomas, 1999). Unfortunately Rita's family did not receive the understanding and support necessary to normalize their experience, reinforce family strengths or provide opportunities to grieve. Her parents' denial of the deafness resulted in unrealistic expectations that Rita be able to "hear" by lip-reading. These unrealistic expectations resulted in increased frustration on the part of her parents, and as a consequence Rita felt a sense of sense of badness and failure. The frustration on the part of Rita's mother resulted in labeling Rita's inability to hear as "stubborn." As a consequence, Rita withdrew from this stressful situation by frequently running to her safe haven, "a tree house." This behavior served as a protection from her mother's rejection as well as protected Rita's mother from her own inadequacy as a parent.

At an early age, parents must make major decisions about the educational environment and accommodations for their children. Although

Rita's parents never learned sign language, they selected an educational placement that facilitated manual communication. At the age of four, Rita attended a residential school for the deaf. It was at the school that Rita acquired language (sign language), interacted with her peers and had an opportunity to proceed developmentally in acquiring mastery and competence socially and academically. The school provided the opportunity to socialization and learn cultural norms; thus providing an opportunity to develop a social identity. Language facilitated the ability to relate and engage with others, assist in understanding the world and people in their environment, as well as begin to develop a sense of mastery, identity, and greater self control (Glickman, 1996).

Although children need to develop coping strategies to deal with their differences, the provision of a supportive academic environment for children with disabilities is extremely critical component of their development. Erikson (1950) noted that by the age of five or six, disabled children begin to notice that they are "different." Children who are disabled are vulnerable to internalizing the negative stigmatization. Philosophical approaches to education of children with special needs vary from total integration to separatism such as special schools or programs that focus on a particular need of the child. Educational opportunities for deaf children include mainstream programs, self contained classrooms, private schools as well as special schools for deaf children. Regardless of the philosophical/structural framework, individual educators are challenged to include specific educational accommodations for children who have disabilities. The development of language gave Rita the opportunity to begin to understand herself and the "world around her." She started to make friends, joined an athletic club and exceled in academics. Rita's achievements were validated at the school. She developed a sense of community and began to develop a positive identity as a deaf person. This experience resulted in the partial externalization of negative introjects related to her deafness as a "bad thing" disability. Equally important she met a deaf teacher who convinced her that she would be able to go to college and be a "productive" member of society. Fortunately, the Deaf community helped Rita externalize some of the negative introjects that were internalized not only by society, but more importantly by her family who denied her deafness, thus rejecting a significant part of her being.

Mackelprang and Salsgiver (1999) emphasize the importance of exposure to peer and role models who have disabilities. Richie, Ferfuson, Gomez, El-Khoury, and Adamalys' (2003) research on landmine survivors who experienced a loss a limb suggest that "Staying connected to others is important to our healthier survivors. More specifically, our survivors talked about the importance of peer support, of the role models that other rehabilitated amputees can play" (p. 35).

Young adulthood focuses on preparation for a career or occupation. The transition to adulthood/to the work environment and training may be more stressful for those individuals who have a disability. One's self esteem is contingent on one's ability to perform with competence in some area, to feel a sense of belonging with some social peer group or recognize that "difference" is not negative. This integral relationship between financial security, independence, and self competence depends on the ability of the work environment to provide appropriate accommodations, hire individuals who are disabled as well as provide an opportunity for social contact.

Rita was fortunate to go to a college that provided accessible communication to deaf individuals. After college, she became a professional in the Deaf community. She married a deaf man and had two hearing children. The deaf community offered a refuge from the discrimination and barriers to communication in the hearing world. Rita was fortunate to be able to meet many of her developmental needs within this community. However, there was some residual affect related to her parents "rejection" of her deafness. Rita had difficulty trusting hearing people, idealized her hearing children, and continued to harbor some feelings of inadequacy and resentment.

SOCIAL WORK INTERVENTIONS

Children depend on their families for a sense of security and support. The importance of secure attachment for children with their caregivers is closely related to the child's ability to trust, achieve competence and developing coping strategies against stress. Attachment with parents may be greatly affected by unresolved grief related to the disability. Although the attachment process is dynamic (the parent-child relationship changes over time), Rita's parents were unable to adjust to the deafness, but resulting in neglect and rejection. Individuals who experience continual discrimination and rejection may require additional time to develop a rapport with the social worker. This holding environment includes an ability to provide unconditional regard and support, minimizing the expectations of the client.

When Rita entered treatment, she had a serious drinking problem. She complained of frequent altercations with her husband and children.

Although Rita's complaints were valid, a majority of the beginning stages of intervention focused on the relationship between the social worker and the client; focusing on issues of trust and an ability to be an empathic listener:

> T: *Rita you had unrealistic expectations placed on you all your life. You were expected to hear.*
> R: *I'm not comfortable with this.*
> T: *It's difficult for you to believe that someone could accept you for you.*

Clients who feel different frequently experience the process of "not being understood." Validation, empathy and unconditional regard are core elements to the healing process, thus the social worker must be vigilant to provide a "holding environment" for an a considerable amount of time (Cohen, 2000). The externalization of negative introjects that were internalized from significant others is a major component of the work. Clients who have internalized a bad representation of self must be able to explore the origins of these representations. The social worker must be aware of the transference, countertransference and intersubjective processes in order to help organize, interpret and analyze the process.

For many months Rita complained that I looked angry at her. Exploring and validating her perceptions were a crucial component of "starting where the client is at" and feeling understood. However, it was equally important to share the intersubjective process, the social worker's feeling and perceptions that contradicted Rita's perceptions. Many times Rita's perceptions were influenced by the transferences related to her critical and angry mother. Once this component was brought to her awareness, the opportunity to grieve and mourn the parents "she never had" and to recognize their limitations, she was able to externalize the internalized negativism.

The Deaf community helped Rita externalize some of the negative discrimination of society. The process of externalizing the negative introjects internalized from her family of origin required several years of work. The work focused on the transferential process, becoming aware of the pain and hurt by her parents and beginning to grieve her lost childhood, not the disability per se but that fact that she did not have a supportive family who accepted her. Social work interventions helped Rita gain insight to the inadequacies of her parents which helped shed her own feelings of badness. Additionally, the lack of communication resulted in traumatic experiences of confusion, feelings of abandonment (when left at the school for the deaf) and anxiety. Interventions focused on resolution of the reenactments of painful silences and experiences as a young child. Through this process, Rita was able to get in touch with unresolved feelings of anxiety, fear, loneliness and anger in order gain control of her past and be able to move on:

T: *What feeling do you have when you look at pictures of your mother?*
R: *Well, I don't know. I was never really attached to my mother. She told me she loved me before she died, but I didn't believe her . . . well . . . in fact I was not trusting because I never knew her . . . and she never knew me. There is a depth . . . a sharing of feelings that I have with my daughters. I never had that with my mother. I wish things could be different . . . she told me she wished I could hear. I never asked her what she meant.*
T: *What did it mean to you?*
R: *It meant not accepting me as a whole person . . . not knowing me as a person. That I am different and that she felt something was wrong with who I am. My family never understood me.*

When parents deny the disability of their child, they are not accepting an integral part of their child; not accepting that their children can be different and have different needs. For individuals who were born with a disability or who acquired a disability at an early age may have the addition challenge of dealing with parental attitudes that may have been internalized at a young age. Parents' denial may result in failures to make appropriate accommodations for special needs. The inability to meet the developmental needs of a child may result in feelings of being rejected or in fact over protection which sends the laden message that the child is not capable of performing thus interfering with a sense of competence and mastery.

DISCUSSION

The integration of a multidimensional approach to interventions in work with individuals is essential. From a biological/medical perspective it is important to understand the multifactorial relationship of disability; one must consider the onset of the disability, the age of the individual, the course of the condition (progressive vs. stable), the type of disability, as well as the functional limitations that are caused by the condition. The birth of a child with a disability presents specific developmental challenges and adaptations. The interactional process between caregiver and baby is essential to support the developmental tasks related to mobility, exploration of the environment, babbling, social skills as well as the development of trust. The time frames to achieve certain developmental tasks may differ and children with disabilities may need special accommodations to achieve specific landmarks.

Of significant importance is an understanding of the disability and the accommodations necessary to facilitate the maturation process. Realistic expectations are a key factor to the achievement of mastery in the areas of physical, social and cognitive development. A parent, for example, who does not have realistic understanding of the abilities of their infant, may become frustrated when their infant does not respond as expected. Assessment of the family adaptive processes to a child with special needs is essential in order to understand the financial resources, time, flexibility of family roles, as well as the family's ability to deal with stress by constructive communication and problem solving. Previous family functioning as it relates to coping with loss and developmental challenges may be beneficial to the assessment process. Families need opportunities to grieve and to adjust to the loss (Marsh & Johnson, 1999). They must create a balance between doing too much and doing too little. Psycho-education may assist the family in acquiring a realistic understanding of a child's abilities as well as learn the specific skills necessary to facilitate the child's development. Families who do not have social, educational or community support may have more difficulty in coping with stress. Quite often social workers are overwhelmed by the challenges of the disability, ignoring the individual and familial needs. Crucial to family intervention is the ability to address not only the special needs of the family member who is disabled but to support and encourage family members' individual interests, goals and needs. Families need to have fun together, have opportunities to be a couple and siblings need to have family support in addressing their own individual needs and desires as well. The social construction of deafness as a disability is one dimensional (Cohen, 2000). Families and individuals alike must challenge the social discrimination laden in the meaning of disabilities. Equally important is an understanding of the multiple/ diverse adaptations of the individual within a specific social context. The availability of resources is a crucial component of the adaptation process. For Rita, the Deaf community provided an avenue to develop a social identity as a deaf individual, partially challenging the negative stigma of deafness as well as providing Rita with an environment in which her strengths were validated and her abilities cultivated. However, systemic issues are quite complex (Harvey, 1989). Educational resources are only one of many systems that are involved with children who have disabilities. Quite often health and medical resources including the availability of organ transports and rehabilitation services are necessary. The advent of technology has greatly enhanced medical care, rehabilitation services and adaptive devices such as laser treatment for blindness, cochlear implant for deafness, power wheelchairs, auditory books and so forth. Accessibility for affordable home care, protective environments, religious and social institutions and support groups are equally important. Social workers should modify their approaches and select interventions that are ego/socially syntonic with the client's strengths, abilities, and culture.

CHALLENGES OF HAVING A SPINAL CORD INJURY: THE CASE OF LAUREEN

According to Quinn (1998) approximately 200,000 individuals in the United States experience a spinal cord injury. Approximately two-thirds of those who acquire a spinal cord injury, do so before the age of 30. The degree of injury or the extent to which the spinal cord is severed will determine the severity of paralysis. Usually an injury above the C3 requires assistance with breathing and may result in death. A vertebrae C7 injury, for example, usually entails paralysis of the arms and legs. A lesion may be complete or partial; individuals with an injury of the C7 level may be able to retain some arm and/or hand functions. Quadriplegia entails injury to all limbs; paraplegia results in paralysis to the lower body and may involve the lower back (lumbar), chest (thoracic) or sacral (tailbone). Sacral or lumbar injuries may entail loss of bladder or bowel control.

Subsequent to the injury, individuals must obtain medical care in order to stabilize the vertebral column (Spoltore & O'Brien, 1995). The individual may be confined to a frame that attempts to prevent ulcers or pressure sores and helps to enhance circulation. Medical concerns include autonomic dysreflexia which involves blood pressure and pulse rate, pressure ulcers (decubitus), and urinary tract infections. If there is pressure on the spinal cord or nerve roots, surgery such as decompressive laminectomy or a spinal fusion may be indicated. On February 18, 1977, Laureen, an eighteen-year-old who recently graduated high school was on the way to a club with her boyfriend when a horse crossing a four way highway jumped on their car causing the car to crash into a telephone pole. Laureen sustained serious spinal cord injuries resulting in quadriplegia at the C 5-6 level. She reports, "It was like a death . . . it was like starting life all over again." The injury affected all aspects of her life: individual and sexual identity, independence and self care, finances, career goals and employment, medical care and health, family life, social life, as well as her future goals. Initially, Laureen underwent surgery (lamenectomy) that involved a cervical fusion, taking a bone from her hip to fuse in the cervical region of her neck. Fifty-five pound tongs were drilled into the top of her skull to stabilize her neck so it would heal properly. Initially, a body cast was necessary in order to be able to sit. The pain was so severe, pain medication was indicated.

"Starting all over again" as Laureen frequently remarked entailed dealing with traumatic losses in order to get acquainted with her body and re-learn how to perform necessary daily activities of living. Bodily functions such as voiding and defecation required attention. In order to prevent urinary tract infections and decubitus, special attention focused on her diet and supplementary intake of vitamins as well as conscious efforts to move in order to prevent this skin irritation/condition. Her multiple surgeries included surgery to alleviate the tethering of her spinal cord, decades after her injury. Laureen had to understand her new bodily needs, re-learn how to perform daily tasks of living, such as personal care (dressing, bathing, feeding, eliminations of her bladder and bowels) and learn how to perform activities requiring mobility and travel. It also required dependency on others. Laureen had personal aides that helped her with much of her personal care: bath, dress, transfer from her bed into a power wheelchair as well as assist with her catheter and help her evacuate her bowels.

ADJUSTMENT:
INTERNAL AND EXTERNAL LOCUS OF CONTROL

Professionals specializing in behavioral sciences discuss both the internal and external locus of control. The internal processes incorporate the psychological adjustment and are contingent on one's pre-morbid personality traits and the interrelationship with adjustment related to one's identity; body functions and changes that occur as a consequence of the injury. The external locus of control involves the loss of status and privileges, employment, social, and recreational opportunities contingent on the accessibility of resources. The interrelationship between the internal and external locus of control is vital in understanding the adjustment process.

Initial Trauma

Immediately after her accident, Laureen was in a state of shock. After coming out of a coma and beginning to realize that she could not move, Laureen described her feelings:

> I was scared, depressed, angry, and unsure of everything. I became dependent on people for every aspect of my life. My survival was dependent on others and I hated it. In the hospital, my food tray was always cold because I had to wait for someone to feed me. I remember depending on a nurse to feed me in the hospital and my food was always cold.

Laureen described herself as a typical teenager. She had a boyfriend, planned to go to college and was working part time to support her future goals. Her dreams were shattered; the traumatic losses affected every aspect of her young life:

> You know I'm an introvert and I lost my privacy. Strangers and family alike saw my nude body . . . I felt demoralized and humiliated.

> Dealing with this disability is a constant struggle. If your caretaker not to show up and then you are stuck in bed all day and can't do anything.

Trauma, loss, and crisis theory are applicable to those individuals who sustain severe disabilities or injuries (Keany & Glueckauf, 1999, Richie, Ferguson, Gomez, El-Khoury, & Adamaly, 2003). Crucial to the adjustment of a traumatic loss, is the social workers respect for the protective and defensive structures that are intact while individuals deal with trauma on a sub or unconscious level. Clearly this means that social workers should make assessments related to the strengths and weaknesses of the individual's premorbid personality in order to help facilitate the adjustment process. Dealing with the trauma of the injury is both internal and external. Laureen stated:

> Social workers need to understand that the changes are both internal and external. Of course the advent of ADA helped us out, but

you need to understand that I felt helpless . . . it was like a death. I had to relearn EVERYTHING. I had to get reacquainted with my body . . . find out what I could and could not do. I had to pay special attention to my functions, my skin, my diet, my medical conditions. . . . (Laureen, 2004)

The foundation of social work practice encompasses the interrelationship between individuals/families/groups and their environment. Galvin and Hons (2003) stated, ". . . the deep inner suffering that results from oppression is not an individual response to personal tragedy but is as much a social problem as lack of access to public spaces, discrimination in the workplace and the denial of resources necessary for independent living (Corker, 1998; Morris, 1991; Thomas, 1999, p. 49). The oppression includes limited access to adequate health care, housing, education, religious, employment, and social and public resources. The application of an ecological framework to social work assessment and practice is crucial to the understanding of disabilities throughout the generations. Perhaps the following example exemplifies the limited access and discrimination of the 1970s:

I remember having to go to court. You won't believe this, but my father had to carry me up the stairs of the court room because there were no ramps in the early 1980s. I remember staying home most of the time. I guess I understand in some ways why my parents overprotected me. (Laureen, 2004)

The advent of ADA helped disabled individuals become more independent related to the tasks of daily living as well as began to address discrimination in the work and educational fields. However, Laureen was not able to fulfill her career dreams:

After completing two years of college, I wanted to continue my education. I would have liked to study art history and work in fine art museums. The universities were too far from where I lived. Living in the dorm was not an option since there were not sufficient accommodations for my disability. I depended on my aging father to take me to school, the stores, the doctors . . . furthering my education at that time was not an option.

Discrimination not only prevented Laureen from pursuing her education but she was not able to keep the employment she did secure. "I was slow or the boss would not permit me to take sick leave when necessary."

In addition to inaccessibility to many resources, financial considerations are paramount. Financial considerations are not only limited to medical care but include the accommodations necessary to live as independently as possible. This may include motorized wheel chairs and scooters, lifts in vans, utensils, special stoves and beds, i.e., Structural accommodations include wider entrances to buildings and rooms; showers to accommodate a wheelchair, special door knobs, stoves and sinks faucets and light switches that are able to be reached in a wheelchair. Repairs for broken chair lifts in one's van, wheelchair problems and mechanical repairs due to wear and age should be taken into account. In addition, personal aides may be financially costly. Laureen and her partner, John, hire a personal aide to help them five hours a day. The aide comes in the morning to help them with personal care; bathing, grooming and transfers to their power wheelchair as well as the evening to help situate them for bed. Laureen described this dilemma:

> You know having a personal aide is a challenge in and of itself. Let me describe a "bad" day. Saturday morning around 6:10 I received a call from my aide saying that she wasn't coming due to a "vertigo" spell. Well, it just so happened that Thursday was her birthday and her live-in boyfriend celebrated Friday evening and she suffered from, "having too much of a good time." Vertigo hmmmm. . . . I can't stand it. John and I have to contend with this EVERY DAY. We tried to ask another aide for help but she was not available. I wanted to say *screw it* and stay in bed all day, but John called his 72 year old mother to help us out. I hate that she has to help in this way . . . my urinary bag (which leaked) needed to be connected, she dressed me . . . how embarrassing . . . (Laureen, 2004)

The problem of securing a competent and caring personal care assistant is a challenge for many individuals who are disabled. Laureen's friend, an individual who has quadriplegia, decided to set up a Website to list aide that are competent as well as those who are incompetent, do not show up, take advantage by borrowing and never pay back and/or show insensitivity to their clients.

The Social Construction of Disability

One cannot separate the psychological adjustments from the contextual environment. As stated previously the social construction of disability is powerful. Galvin and Hons (2003) state:

In semiotic terms, the signifier, "disabled" becomes attached to a range of significatory concepts such as weak, passive, dependent, unintelligient, worthless and problematic, so that when the word is spoken, a negative, even partially subconscious, feeling is evoked (p. 55).

Laureen frequently discussed the stereotyping as preventing people from getting to know her:

Some people see me as if I have no brain since I'm in a wheelchair. Its almost like it's my responsibility to prove to the public that I can function carry on a normal conversation, and that my physical disability is not a mental one. People see the wheelchair and make those assumptions. If people could look beyond the chair and see me for who I am, I think people would realize that folks with disabilities are really quite normal. Society places such a high priority on looks. There is this fear... as if I'm retarded or as if others will "catch" what I have. I chalk it up to ignorance.

Individuals with disabilities have to not only content with the social construction of disability and environmental responses, but they need to challenge these labels and externalize the negative introjects that they may have internalized.

Adjustment

The process of adaptation and adjustment Livneh and Antonak, (1990) may include but are not limited to the following reactions of shock, anxiety, denial, depression, internalized and externalized anger, acknowledgment, and adjustment. In addition, as stated previously individuals need to challenge the negative labels and status related to the meaning and treatment of disability in this society. Shock may take various forms such as psychological numbness, disorganization or depersonalization; anxiety may consist of panic, flooding, or confusion. The anxiety may be related to issues of survival and safety as well as the risk of doing tasks for oneself or in fact depending on others for meeting one's essential needs. Denial involves unrealistic understanding of the long range consequences of the disability; depression involves feelings of hopelessness, helplessness, low self esteem, and loss of purpose. Although depression is common and a "typical" response to the magnitude of loss and adjustment required for those who sustain a disability, depression can also constrict one's time perspective related to setting goals for the future (Marz, 2004). Thus one's depression (i.e., depending on the severity, length manifestations) may limit one's options and strategies in coping with one's disability. The process of adjustment may indeed result in different forms of coping. It may mean challenging previous values and life styles, reassessing one's life goals with an appreciation for different life challenges, values and personal growth.

Laureen's Journey Towards Adaptation

Individuals may appear "in denial" however they are working through adjustment and acceptance on an unconscious level; grieving losses and preparing for the major adjustments that will be necessary to daily functioning. Laureen discusses the process of her adjustment:

> I spent the subsequent ten years of my life under the protection of my parents. They were very supportive but over-protective of me... they smothered me! Remember, I sustained my injuries in the 1970s... at that time you really didn't see people outside in wheelchairs. There weren't any accommodations for us.

As previously stated, family response to one's disability has a powerful influence on the individual. Christopher Reeve, the famous actor who was thrown from a horse and subsequently sustained paralysis in 1995 noted the importance of family support during his rehabilitation:

> I was lucky.... Right after the injury she (my wife) said, "you're you and I love you,"...I noticed when I was in rehabilitation that a fellow patient who had good family support and loving relationships did better than another fellow patient whose personal life was more chaotic and troubled. (2003, p. 82)

Laureen's family responses proved to be mixed; the tremendous love and support helped her cope but their overprotectiveness resulted in a period of time of complete dependency. Dealing with the multiple losses resulted in not only depression but anger at what happened to her. Lane (1999) notes that "...anger of people with disabilities is rarely understood or accepted as valid or necessary" (p. 174). She expatiates on this topic; "It is our ability to experience anger which allows us to experience love, joy, and deep caring for life" (p. 173). Anger is clearly part of the grief process, the actual losses as well as those imposed by society and the lack of equal access. In times of overwhelming loss, some individuals may harbor self directed bitterness or excessive guilt usually the result of internalized anger. Laureen externalized some of her anger, having temper outbursts directed at her mother. On the other hand, Laureen was aware that she has internalized some of the negative labeling imposed by society, "Sometimes I don't feel like a person...like I'm unimportant...a second class citizen." Internalized anger may result in depression. Laureen spent the first decade of her life under the protection of her parents; she was too anxious and depressed to pursue any interests. She assumed she would live under her parents protection for the rest of her life. When Laureen was in her early 30s she realized that her parents may die before her. Acknowledgment of one's disability usually focuses on the cognitive knowledge whereas adjustment focuses on the integration of behavior and cognition. Perhaps the impetus for making major adaptations was related to Laureen's concern for her future; the fact that she could not depend on her parents for the rest of her life. Laureen enrolled in a rehabilitation program. She was realistic about many of her functional limitations by the time of her enrollment in a rehabilitation program. Physically she was stronger and she began using assistive devises to help her with her independent skills. For example she began to use a quad knife (a serrated knife that has a cuff that slips around the palm the hand), a cutting board that has two nails drilled into the board to keep the food stationary so that she could cut food, pots and pans that have special handles and lids so she could easily open the pot covers and pick up the pots, special typing aids that slip over her palm help her type, use the calculator to press the number buttons and also make turning pages in a book easier.

The adjustment process is a continuous struggle. Individuals are challenged by the social constructions of disability, which may include a shift in their own values and perceptions (Kelly, Keany, & Glueckauf, 1999). Individuals may focus on an internal and spiritual life, others search for a sense of belonging and many combine both internal and external factors.

Theorists in the field of object relations such as Mahler, Pine and Bergman (1975) discuss the importance of not only a sense of individual identify but a sense of attachment with others (Goldstein, 1995). In particular Kohut (1971) discussed the importance of a sense of humanness, likeness to, and partnership with others (Goldstein, 1995). Laureen's involvement in the Disability community helped the adjustment process. Not only did Laureen go back to school to obtain an associate degree, she met her partner through the internet. This relationship, sense of comradeship and connectiveness was a crucial component to her adjustment, adding meaning and happiness to her life.

SUMMARY

Theorists in the field of disability (Harvey, 1989; Corker, 1995, Quinn, 1990) note the importance of diverse processes in one's struggle to accept one's disability. Clearly the readjustment entails relearning and understanding of one's "new" persona." This means letting go of the person one once was and learning and figuring out who one is. Keany and Glueckauf (1999) emphasis the integration of loss theory as part of the adaptation process. The "relearning of oneself" may necessitate challenging or broadening one's scope of values as well as subordination of others such as the value of physique. Theorists such as Elliott, Uswatte, Lewis and Palmatier (2000) discuss the importance of finding meaning and purpose in life. In many cases, this means a shift in one's orientation and values. Some individuals become more focused on an internal life (spiritual life) not only to help heal and give meaning to one's life, but to challenge the external values of physical appearance and pleasures which may be too difficult to obtain as an individual with a physical disability. The value changes that are strongly related to acceptance relate to acceptance of the disability as nondevaluating (Keany & Glueckauf, 1999). Laureen's adaptations focused on the ability to find out who she became, to relearn how her body functioned as well as her functional limitations so she could at least challenge or learn how to overcome them. This self discovery included going to back to college, obtaining employment and more importantly finding a mate who she could spend the rest of her life with. Her soul mate, John who also acquired a spinal cord injury has been her role model and mentor. The process of adjustment began a long time ago when Laureen realized that she would have to fight in a way she never had done; that her parents would not be able to take care of her forever. Laureen ended her story with the words, "I'm coming back . . . although I withdrew many years, I'm Laureen again" One's meaning in life and contributions may take on many forms. Underlying the desire to change requires a supportive network; family, friends and or the disability community and professionals.

DISABILITY AND SOCIAL WORK EDUCATION

Values

Values and ethics are one of the most important foundations in social work practice. Although social workers may have good intentions, quite often they are challenged to understand diversity; different life styles, cultures, experiences as perceptions of the world and value systems. Many times social workers are unaware of their values or the stereotypical perceptions they have of disability. Mackelprang and Salsgiver (1990) emphasize the need to address the prejudices and stereotypes that professionals bring to their practice. Empathic failures by the therapist (Cohen, 2000) in work with individuals who were deaf were primary due to the lack of knowledge of deafness and unawareness of the social workers value system and its impact on the social work relationship (countertransference). Accurate assessment and ongoing intervention necessitates an empathic understanding of the client's life situation. Social work students are challenged to use their knowledge of oppression and diversity in the development of an empathic understanding of client situations.

Knowledge

The ecological and system framework provides a comprehensive understanding of the client/environment situation. This framework includes the physical/medical/developmental/interpersonal/social/political processes that are involved with the adaptation process. In the case of both Rita and Laureen, great emphasis was placed on attitudes towards those with disabilities. These attitudes have great influence not only interpersonal relations but impact on policy and civil rights. Technological advances, current political values and policies impact one's human rights and have clearly played a significant role in the lives of those who are disabled. As we listen to the life stories and struggles of clients who have disabilities, we gain knowledge into their internal and external world and daily challenges. Paying attention to the life narratives of clients augment competency and result in a continuation of the development of knowledge and enhancement of skills. Within the ecological and systemic framework, social workers make assessments, integrating the multiple influences of the "client in environmental" match in order to facilitate the adaptation processes. Social workers are not expected to understand the integral aspects of every disability, however they should be cognizant of gaps in their knowledge and continue the self learning process.

Skill

As stated previously, a positive alliance with clients include an ability to communicate, an understanding of the client's diverse life style and values as well as be sensitive to the client's struggles and modes of adaptation. This skill involves an understanding of one's own values and as well as a tendency to be aware of one's own countertransferences as they relate to the client/social work relationship. This awareness will facilitate a better appreciate of client values, strengths and both the intrapsychic and external challenges for their clients. Theories that provide a sense of empowerment may include but are not limited to crisis intervention, grief work, family therapy, narrative treatment, advocacy and community organization. Sensitivity to the multiple oppressive forces will enhance one's understanding of the client dilemma as well as be a crucial in the development of interventions that facilitate the healing process. Perhaps adaptation of a disability is one of the most significant challenges in life. Bach (1977) says, "An easy life doesn't teach us anything. In the end, it's the learning that matters; what we've learned and how we've grown" (p. 110). Bach's perspective is important for both clients and social workers alike. As social workers we need to continue our journey of learning.

REFERENCES

Bach, R. (1977). *Illusions*. New York: Creative Enterprises, Inc.
Cohen, C. (2001). *Individual psychotherapy with deaf and hard of hearing individuals: Perceptions of the consumer.* Unpublished doctoral dissertation. Smith College: Northampton, MA.
Cohen, C. (2003). Psychotherapy with deaf and hard of hearing individuals: Perceptions of the consumer. *Journal of Social Work in Disability & Rehabilitation, 2*(2/3) 23-46.

Corker, M. (1998). Disability discourse in a postmodern world. In T. Shakespeare (Ed), *The disability reader: Social science perspectives* (pp. 221-233). London: Continuum.

Elliott, T., Uswatte, G., Lewis, L., & Palmatier, A. (2000). Goal instability and adjustment to physical disability. *Journal of Counseling Psychology, 47*(2) 251-265.

Elson, M. (1986). *Self psychology in clinical social work.* New York: Norton Publishers.

Erikson, E. (1950). *Childhood and society.* New York: Norton Press.

Gallagher, C. K., & Hough, S. (2001). Ethnicity and age issues: Attitudes affecting rehabilitation of individuals with spinal cord injury. *Rehabilitation Psychology 46*(3), 312-321.

Galvin, R., & Hons, B. A. (2003). The making of a disabled identity: A linguistic analysis of marginalization. *Disability Studies Quarterly, 23*(2), 49-70.

Glickman, N. (1996). What is culturally affirmative psychotherapy? In N. Glickman & M. Harvey (Eds.), *Culturally affirmative psychotherapy with deaf persons* (pp. 1-57). Mahwah, NJ: Lawrence Erlbaum Associates, Publishers.

Goldstein, E. (1995). *Ego psychology and social work practice.* New York: Free Press.

Harvey, M. (1989). *Psychotherapy with deaf and hard of hearing persons: A systemic model.* Mahwah, NJ: Lawrence Erlbaum Associates, Publishers.

Hueber, R., & Thomas, K. (1999). The relationship between attachment, psychotherapy and childhood disability. In R. Marinelli & A. Dell Orto (Eds.), *The psychological and social impact of disability* (pp. 67-85). New York: Springer Publishing Co.

Keany, K., & Glueckauf, R. (1999). Disability and value change: An overview and reanalysis of acceptance of loss theory. In R. Marinelli & A. Dell Orto (Eds.), *The psychological and social impact of disability* (pp. 139-151). New York: Springer Publishing Co.

Kohut, H. (1971). *The analysis of the self.* New York: International University Press.

Lane, N. (1999). A theology of anger when living with disability. In R. Marinelli & A. Dell Orto (Eds.), *The psychological and social impact of disability* (pp. 173-186). New York: Springer Publishing Co.

Mackelprang, R., & Salsgiver, R. (1999). *Disability: A diversity model approach in human service practice.* Pacific Grove, CA: Brooks/Cole Publishing Co.

Mahler, M., Pine, F., & Bergman, N. (1975). *The psychological birth of the human infant.* New York: Basic Books.

Marschark, M. (1993). *Psychological development of deaf children.* New York: Oxford University Press.

Marsh, D., & Johnson, D. (1999). The family experience of mental illness: Implications for intervention. In R. Martinelli & A. Dell Orto (Eds.), *The psychological and social impact of disability* (pp. 340-357). New York: Springler Publishing Co.

Martz, E. (2004). Do reactions of adaptation to disability influence the fluctuation of future time orientation among individuals with spinal cord injury? *Rehabilitation Bulletin, 47*(2) 86-98.

Piazza, K. (2003). Commentary. *The Exceptional Parent, 33*(7), 76.

Powell, L. H., Shahabi, L., & Thoreson, C. E. (2003). Religion and spirituality: Linkages to physical health. *American Psycholoist, 58*(1), 36-52.

Quinn, P. (1998). *Understanding disability: A lifespan approach.* Thousand Oaks, CA: Sage Publications.

Reeve, C., & Allen, C. (2003). One finger at a time. *Psychology Today, 36*(2), 82.

Richie, B. S., Ferguson, A., Gomez, M., El-Khoury, D., & Adamaly, Z. (2003). Resilience in survivors of traumatic limb loss. *Disability Studies Quarterly 23*(2), 29-41.

Sandvin, J. T. (2003). Loosening the bonds and changing identities: Growing up with impairments in post-war Norway. *Disability Studies Quarterly, 23*(20), 5-19.

Schlesinger, H. (1978). *At home among strangers.* Washington, DC: Gallaudet University Press.

Solomon, L., Springer, S., & Vachon, M. (1993). Disordered communication in deaf family members. *Family Process, 32*, 171-183.

Spoltore, T. A., & O'Brien, A. M. (1995). Rehabilitation of the spinal cord injured patient. *Orthopaedic Nursing, 14*(3), 7-14.

St. Claire, M. (1996). *Object relations and self psychology.* Monterey, CA: Brooks/Cole Publishing Company.

Thomas, C. (1999). *Female forms: Experiencing and understanding disability.* Buckingham: Open University Press.

Thomas, C. (1999). Narrative identity and the disabled self. In M. Corker & S. French (Eds.), *Disability Discourse* (pp. 39-47). Buckingham: Open University Press.

Thompson, C. E. (1990). Transition of the disabled adolescent to adulthood. *Pediatrician, 17*, 308-313.

Thompson, N. J., Coker, J., Krause, J. S., & Henry, E. (2003). Purpose of life as a mediator of adjustment after spinal cord injury. *Rehabilitation Psychology, 48*(2),100-108.

doi:10.1300/J198v06n01_08

The Impact of Sight Loss in Social Work Practice

Cathy Orzolek-Kronner

SUMMARY. This article intends to familiarize the social worker with the various definitions of blindness and sight loss, common obstacles faced by persons with sight loss, general therapeutic issues, when and how to use self-disclosure of a disability, and the ways in which the social worker can use his or her disability, specifically sight-loss, as an instrumental therapeutic tool with clients. Case examples will be provided to illustrate effective interventions and the various ways in which a disability may impact a client or clients. In addition, a brief discussion of various theoretical approaches to understanding disabilities is outlined. doi:10.1300/J198v06n01_09 *[Article copies available for a fee from The Haworth Document Delivery Service: 1-800-HAWORTH. E-mail address: <docdelivery@haworthpress.com> Website: <http://www.HaworthPress.com> © 2007 by The Haworth Press, Inc. All rights reserved.]*

KEYWORDS. Vision loss, social worker with a disability, use of professional self, psychodynamic theory

Cathy Orzolek-Kronner, PhD, LCSW, is Assistant Professor and Program Director, Department of Social Work, McDaniel College, Westminster, MD 21157-4390 USA (E-mail: corzolek@mcdaniel.edu).

[Haworth co-indexing entry note]: "The Impact of Sight Loss in Social Work Practice." Orzolek-Kronner, Cathy. Co-published simultaneously in *Journal of Social Work in Disability & Rehabilitation* (The Haworth Press, Inc.) Vol. 6, No. 1/2, 2007, pp. 157-177; and: *Disability and Social Work Education: Practice and Policy Issues* (ed: Francis K. O. Yuen, Carol B. Cohen, and Kristine Tower) The Haworth Press, Inc., 2007, pp. 157-177. Single or multiple copies of this article are available for a fee from The Haworth Document Delivery Service [1-800-HAWORTH, 9:00 a.m. - 5:00 p.m. (EST). E-mail address: docdelivery@haworthpress.com].

INTRODUCTION

If you could only see how fat I am, then you would know why I cannot allow myself to eat.

This explanation or some version of it, was commonly given to me by the clients I worked with in individual counseling and group therapy. They had eating problems such as anorexia nervosa, and bulimia nervosa and I had an eye disease that significantly compromised my vision. Initially in treatment, many of my clients would suggest that they doubted I could help them because I could not "accurately see the burden of her fat body." I would always suggest that there were no guarantees, but I could try to understand the weight of her being if she could begin to describe herself to me both externally and internally (the inner self, which neither of us could really see).

Clients would usually begin with long and detailed descriptions of their outer selves using such words as "disgusting, gross, flabby, repulsive, and revolting" to describe various features of their outward appearance. These same clients were generally at a loss when it came to defining their inner selves. For example, I would often explain to Jane that I was finding it difficult to understand her in a whole way, but it seemed that this too was true of her. I would also reflect to Jane that her external definition of self made it sound as if I was sitting in the room with a monster, yet intuitively I did not get this impression, nor did I feel afraid. These beginnings with the client, in which I revealed a powerful bit of my true self (my low vision and my experience of her), set the foundation for a trusting relationship that would be necessary for Jane's discovery of her whole self and the gains and losses she would ultimately experience in the attainment of that personal insight. Self-discovery and understanding will unfold as paramount themes throughout this article.

BLINDNESS AND LOW VISION

Vision is a complex sense, encompassing the capacity to perceive detail (activity, color, and contrast), and to distinguish objects (Vision Connections, 2004). While these abilities can naturally diminish with age, vision can also be affected by various birth complications, genetic conditions, eye disease, illnesses that can secondarily impact vision such as diabetes, accidents, imposed injury from another, and self-injurious behavior. In some rare cases medications and surgery have led to vision loss as well as poor health and nutrition.

If one experiences a total loss of vision, the result is blindness. While medical advances are profound today, total blindness is almost always a life-long circumstance. In the United States, the term "legal blindness" is commonly used and is characterized by visual acuity of 20/200 or less in the better eye (Wahl, Schilling, Osald, & Heyl, 1999). Corrective lenses or glasses can help some individuals, who are legally blind, while others cannot be helped. If one experiences a partial loss of vision, the result is called low vision, partial visual loss, visual-impairment or sight-impairment. Other persons will have constructed their own terminology for describing their vision or change in vision such as "bad eyes, poor vision, or visually challenged."

It is important to remember that vision can vary from person to person, as does the severity of vision loss. It is helpful to both the client and social worker to have some understanding of the biological, psychological, and sociological aspects of one's visual challenges. It is noteworthy, however, to mention that sometimes the client does not have much understanding of his/her own visual loss as some conditions are extremely complicated, and one's visual field can change on a moment by moment basis (Hyman, 2003).

FUNCTIONAL LIMITATIONS

In order to provide the highest quality of service to persons, who are blind or visually impaired, social workers should be cognizant of some of the barriers or situations their clients may encounter. These issues may include a client's inability to read standard print. Sometimes large print can accommodate a person with low vision and sometimes not. Some people with sight-impairments prefer that instructional material be read to them while others prefer to read it with their own magnification device. Remember that upon most initial meetings paperwork is involved, and thus, the knowledgeable social worker will ask his/her client to identify his/her preference.

People with significant sight loss usually do not drive automobiles. Getting to and from places involves careful planning for someone with a visual challenge. In fact, too often the visually-impaired person who could benefit from counseling or other social work services is denied them based on the absence of transportation or other problems with mobility (Harsh, 1993). If the client identified his/her disability when arranging the initial meeting, the social worker should ask how he/she will be traveling (bus, taxi, accompanied by someone, etc.), and discuss explicit directions to the office from the location in which he/she will be arriving. It is ideal if they social worker can meet his/her new client at a major entrance to the building if his/her office or agency exists within the construct of a larger facility. The social worker must also keep in mind that tardiness for an appointment may be the consequence of public transportation or one's driver rather than client ambivalence. This issue should be explored as both situations have therapeutic value. For example, lateness due to environmental conditions can often evoke feelings of frustration, anger, and the continual reminder of one's dependency on others for survival.

The well-informed social worker must also remember that the client with low vision may not always recognize a familiar face, and it is important to make your presence known to your client. For example, if you meet your client in a waiting room, go up to her and say hello Ms. J., it's _____(your name). There seems to be some tendency for people to speak louder than usual to persons with disabilities. This can be offensive, and the skilled social worker uses his/her regular speaking voice.

Often persons who are totally or partially blind need assistance in walking to the social worker's office. The appropriate method known to persons who have had mobility training is for the sight-impaired person to place his/her hand underneath the elbow of the one who is assisting and walk side by side to the destination. In all circumstances, social workers should be aware of appropriate professional boundaries and implement standard accommodation. Should a client suggest that holding hands would feel less awkward, it is important for the social worker to assert conventional practices, and once in the confidential office explore the origins of the client's request. When working with clients, sighted or unsighted, the implementation of professional ethics and boundaries is essential.

Both institutional and individual discrimination is an obstacle faced by most all persons with disabilities. The repetition of environmental stress, inefficient architecture design, and lack of regard from others can lead to low self-concepts among persons with disabilities (Tam, 1998). In addition, language has a significant impact on the perpetuation of prejudice (Diller, 1999; Morales & Schaefer, 2001). Most social work texts that are used for education and training illuminate the importance of putting the person in front of the disability (i.e., Today, I meet wit Mr. B., a 45-year-old married man who is totally blind). Research has also cautioned effective practitioners not to categorize individuals by the disability (i.e., the blind). Equally important, however, is the social worker's personal choice of words when speaking directly with the client. For example, when initially meeting the client, rather than say, "I am glad to see you made it here." It may be more effective to select words that both parties can relate to or eliminate those words that differentiate the sighted from those with out sight. In other words, a more relational greeting could be, "I'm glad that you made it here."

While these examples may seem trivial in nature, they clearly demonstrate a power differential that sustains an ongoing oppressive attitude both within individuals and the larger society. Most of the time this attitude is out of one's awareness, thus affirming the need for sharp critical thinking skills and personal insight which are two valued aspects of the social work curriculum as recommended by the Council on Social Work Education (CSWE).

CONFRONTING LACK OF KNOWLEDGE AND INSIGHT

A Personal Experience

It has been my experience in a range of roles (social worker, client, professor, student, citizen) that those individuals who are uncomfortable with my visual loss, unconsciously use words directly referring to some aspect of sight far more frequently with me than they do when speaking with persons who are fully sighted. It is always my cue when speaking to new people that if they somehow manage to integrate expressions (in what seems to be out of context), such as "the blind leading the blind, blind alley, blind-sided," etc., within the first five minutes of our conversation, then I know that they are uncomfortable and need to know more about my visual impairment. I typically respond to their cue by weaving my sight-impairment into the conversation. Most of the time, these same people suggest that they are extremely surprised to know this and say such things as "I can't believe it. You do so well," or "Really I thought you were a professor," or better yet, "Oh, do you need some help." Being relatively desensitized to these comments over the years, I usually come back with a witty remark, but each time I hear one of these types of comments, I grow increasingly concerned about the perception people have about persons with disabilities. These types of comments come from persons of all educational levels, classes, creeds, etc. Most of these people by no means intend to be offensive. In fact, it seems they are attempting to communicate some type of sensitive response, yet their good will is underscored by a sentiment of oddity and incapability. The difficulty with this attitude of inferiority seems to be universal and deeply embedded in most people's psyche and is often shared by those who have disabilities themselves. In this way many people who are blind or have low vision have internalize this subjacent attitude and make it their own self-fulfilling prophecy. As a result, our clients with disabilities have few role models and mentors in which to aspire.

A Client's Perspective on the Issue of Discrimination

A few years ago I received a telephone call from a young woman who is totally blind. We had worked together several years prior, but had ended when she eagerly set off to college. She was calling to arrange a couple of therapy visits during her semester break as she felt extremely depressed and was not even sure if she wanted to return to school. I was surprised by this given that only weeks before I had received a short note from her indicating how rewarding college has been. During our first meeting, she recollected a recent conversation with her faculty advisor who she greatly respected. She indicated that last week she met with him to discuss major interest and career options. After listening to her ideas, my client recalled his response.

> Look this is hard for me to say to you because you are such a sweet and bright girl and that's why I don't want you to be disillusioned. The plain and simple fact is, well look around, there's not many blind people out there in careers like you want. Consider computer science. With computer technology today, and the adaptive software you use, you could probably get a good paying job and even work from your home. Make things easy on yourself.

This was devastating to my ambitious, gregarious client who was torn between imagining herself as a lawyer who would later become a judge, and a journalist, which was motivated by her relational self and adventurous disposition. Fortunately my client's ego strength and resiliency drew her out of her depression into a state of anger from which she mobilized herself to return to college, switch advisors, and pursue her passion for the law and constitutional rights.

This may seem to be an inspiring story of remarkable strength, and it is, but equally as significant as the resiliency of my client is the oppressive attitude of the college professor which as his observations suggest, are reinforced by our societal values regarding disability. My hope is that the reader is alarmed by this conversation between the student and her advisor, but, more importantly, willing to examine his/her own values and beliefs around persons with disabilities and their place in this world.

Age as a Freeing Factor to Flexible Thinking

The only demographic characteristic that seems to me to separate people who generally highlight the limitations of people with disabilities from those who do not, is age. Children under approximately age 10 generally consider the possibilities for people to be endless, disability or not. Children also seem to be remarkably creative in identifying alternative ways for people with disabilities to do things. For example, one 5-year-old child who had been referred to me by his pediatrician for some adjustment problems related to his parent's divorce brought in a book and asked me to read it to him. I reminded him that my eyes did not work so well and I could not see the words. He asked me "Can your eyes see the pictures?" I said yes and then he suggested "Well just read the pictures." His idea had greater value then he ever intended because he then realized that he could read the pictures too and consequently felt proud. He later thought of a book he was going to read to his mommy that night, and another that he would take with him to his dad's over the weekend.

Children also offer a refreshing way to view difference. One 8-year-old boy with separation-anxiety once said, "Your lucky, you can always ask to hold someone's hand and nobody thinks your weird." Another young client also saw the good fortune my sight-impairment had for my children (who by the way I had not yet had). "I was thinking your kids are so lucky. I bet you always sit in the front row at the movies. That's where I want to sit but my parents always make us sit in the back."

Finally, children are more inclined to ask questions about what they do not know. Ceconi and Urdang (1994) discuss the candidness of children when working with their social worker who is blind. It is from the child's innocence and natural inquisition that he/she develops a sense of comfort with difference that perhaps may last a lifetime. This study also discusses the utility of a guide dog in working with children.

General Therapeutic Issues

Practitioners often assume that when a client with a disability seeks counseling or other social services it is directly related to the disability, and consequently make the disability a predominant issue. This is not always true (Harsh, 1993). The following exerpt between the client and social worker illustrates this point.

Client: I know you mentioned you had a sight-impairment, but you must have noticed my wheel-chair.

Social Worker: I did.

Client: We've been talking for over 30 minutes and you haven't asked about it. I've been to several different therapists since I've been in this thing and that's always what they ask about first. You know, questions like–How come you're in a wheelchair, Have you always been in a wheelchair, What's it like to be in a wheelchair and on and on.

Social Worker: I can't figure out if you're disappointed I didn't ask, or maybe relieved? I'm not sure what you're trying to tell me.

Client: I guess I'm shocked. It seems to be everybody's focus–well at least the counselor's focus. It seems like the other counselors see my wheelchair as the root of all my problems.

Social Worker: Do you?

Client: No. It's a bad circumstance, but what I never get to talk about is much greater.

Social Worker: So, let's talk about that.

On the other hand, York (1980) warns that it is dangerous to assume that the disability has nothing to do with the problems. He goes on to caution the therapist of not colluding with the client in such a way. The skilled social worker will not disconnect one's disability or deny its existence and the challenges that can be association with it, but rather look for opportunities to explore these issues should the client be encountering resistance.

One may remember that while resistance can impede change, it is often not deliberate and can be unconsciously used to preserve one's self worth. (Goldstein, 1995). The following example provides a look at the social worker's resistance to thoroughly acknowledging the plight of the client in an attempt to simplify the client's reality and make her feel better.

I can't seem to make any of my therapists understand the complexity in communicating my disability to others. I am now working with my fifth counselor and the same thing just happened. I mention the difficulty I have with disclosing my condition to potential romantic partners. I explained to my recent social worker that I cannot find the balance between minimizing the complexity of my condition, and overstating the problems I have in order that I cover it all. This counselor like all the others, gives me the same advice. "Just be honest. If he can't accept it, it's his loss." I always leave feeling despaired. It is my loss and it's not that simple.

This story also serves as an appreciable example of the illusion of social acceptance regarding disabilities. It is an example of repeated attempts by social workers to make the client feel better, when the client is really asking for a safe and secure environment in which to explore her options. Exploring the issue is a fundamental social work skill (Schulman, 1999) and is particularly pertinent to working with people with physical disabilities. Careful exploration of client problems can evoke rich material, cultivate rapport and illicit a sense of confidence in the social worker's capacity to understand and help (Pillari, 2002). In the case above, the social worker may simply ask, "What do you think would be important for your partner to know in the beginning of your relationship?"

If a client seeks the services of a social worker as a direct result of his/her disability, the social worker needs to be equipped with some knowledge of resources, and preferably some knowledge of the disabling condition. While it is appropriate to ask questions pertaining to the disability, it is helpful to the client to have some existing knowledge in order to ask relevant questions. For example, a student intern placed at a community mental health center reported the following experience during a class discussion.

I was observing my supervisor interviewing a new young male client who had multiple sclerosis and was in a wheelchair. He indicated that while he missed playing basketball, he felt fortunate that he was still able to drive. I know my supervisor was just trying to lighten things up but she ended up saying, "well then there's nothing to worry about–It's not like you can go blind from MS." The young man replied in a very sad tone, "Well it's not like I really ever thought about that, but some people do." My supervisor simply said, "Sorry, I didn't know that. I was just making a joke." I was so mad at her. Later she said to me that we can't know everything. I guess she's right in a way, but how much do we need to know as social workers, and how much room is there for not know-ing? I really feel like her ignorance set the client back.

In this scenario another fundamental social work skill was poorly used, timing. Germain and Gitterman (1996) remind us that timing is often the culminating difference between the effective and ineffective generalist social worker. The supervisor unintentionally, yet neverthe-less, evokes another potential loss that the client may not be ready to address. Jokingly, the supervisor brings up "blindness" which turns out to be a potential risk of multiple sclerosis. While disrupting a client's psychological equilibrium can help evoke insight and ultimately benefit the client in insight-oriented psychotherapy, the premature disruption of psychic energy can create severe distress to a client and result in regres-sive behaviors that can sometimes become dehabilitating (Schamess, 1996). While social workers are not expected to be infallible, the best advice to the supervisor in this scenario is to connect only with the con-tent and affect the client brings to the session until a thorough assess-ment is complete. I would caution the supervisor to move beyond her apology and move with the client at his speed.

When a client alludes to a visual loss, all aspects of that loss should be explored. For example, it is important to know when a client expe-rienced the loss, the cause of the loss, and the meaning of the loss to the client. Each of these areas has specific relevance in the client's life. For example, the timing of the sight-loss could evoke radically different issues depending on whether the client was born with the disability or acquired the disability during another life stage (Cohen 2005).

Self-Disclosure and Disability

Upon initially meeting a new client, it has been my experience that acknowledging one's own disability early on in the session puts both client and social worker at greater ease. Beck (1991) also found this to be true for the social worker with a hearing loss. Asch and Rousso (1985) also agree that when disability is part of the characteristics of the therapist, the disability needs to be addressed. In addition, they have found that many people have negative perceptions or uncertainty about the emotional well being, productivity, and capacity to connect to some-one with a disability. They propose that there is substantial evidence to suggest that people without visible disabilities or obvious physical dif-ferences regard people with visible disabilities with a range of emotions that at the very least can affect routine social interactions (Asch & Rousso, 1985).

While disabilities may create therapeutic merit for some clients, there are some situations or disabling conditions that can hinder the therapeutic process or create a therapeutic impasse for others that can only be resolved through a referral to another social work practitioner. While alluded to earlier, it is important to remember conventional communication between client and therapist is usually altered, and needs to be addressed. For example, while we previously discussed some of the benefits to "not being seen," the inability to make appropriate eye contact can be a significant issue and warrants a discussion early on. The absence of this discussion could result in a client feeling like he/she is not being attended to or regarded. In some cases, lack of eye contact could increase the paranoia that often accompanies a psychotic patient. In addition, one's inability to read non-verbal cues, or notice outward signs of affect must be acknowledged. Stating these circumstances in the initial session usually sets a comfortable premise for revisiting these issues when appropriate. For example, on the third session I said to a very shy and depressed 14-year-old girl, "You are particularly quiet today, I bet you wish I could read your face." She signed, "Yes." I then asked her, "Would you be willing to read it to me." She chuckled and said, "Well I would but now its changed." I suggested that she must have turned to the page ahead, but I thought it was important to go back to the previous page and begin reading there.

While I believe that self-disclosure should be used modestly with clients, there are some demographic issues that cannot be overlooked such as age, race, gender, and disability. These factors provide meaningful data which can impede the working alliance or enrich it depending on one's understanding and interpretation of those factors. Other types of self-disclosures may be used more intentionally by the skilled practitioner. In order to be used effectively self-disclosure requires that the social worker be cognizant of his/her personal feelings and thoughts and accepts responsibility for them (Pillar, 2002). While self-disclosures are intended to create a level of mutual understanding and trust between the client and therapist, they can also negatively impact the therapeutic relationship. For instance, some anecdotal client reports infer that identification with the social worker has qualified them for competition with that practitioner. In addition some clients need someone to idealize (Kohut, 1977), rather than identify with and one's sameness can be discouraging rather than encouraging. I would air caution to using one self as an example to clients. If the client is unable to accomplish what you have as an individual who has had barriers to overcome, the client may feel as if he/she has failed. While you may serve as a role model in some cases, never volunteer to be one. Aside from disclosing the disability itself, and how it may impact treatment, the same understanding and utility of self-disclosure should be implemented throughout the helping process.

The Social Worker with a Disability and Effective Intervention

There are many types and degrees of disabilities. This discussion will be limited to physical disabilities specific to sensory and mobility challenges. In accordance with this chapter, the primary focus is on blindness and sight-loss.

While the professional community has been known to raise concerns around the therapeutic effectiveness of social workers with disabilities, some social workers with disabilities have found great therapeutic value in their work with clients when the disability was part of the treatment process (Asch & Rousso, 1985; Beck, 1991; Ceconi & Urdang, 1994). Let us examine an exert from an all female adolescent group therapy meeting on an inpatient hospital unit. Initially, it appears that the social worker's impaired vision had serious repercussions to the group, but as we will later understand paradoxically served as the integral tool that tapped into many repressed client feelings that were necessary to unleash for genuine healing. The therapist gives her account:

The group was more quiet than usual today, It was almost the same group of adolescents who had been meeting each day since last week. Julie just joined the group yesterday, but everyone else was familiar. "What's going on?" I asked. "You all are unusually quite." A moment of silence passed again. "Nancy is cutting herself," blurted out Debra. "Is this true Nancy?," I asked. No response, as someone else in the group squeaked softly, "It is." I got up and escorted Nancy to the nurse's station. The nurses managed Nancy, and I returned to the group. No one said a word. "Can we talk about what just happened?," I asked. No one said a word. I waited patiently. About 10 minutes later Debra said, "Nancy's going to hate me now. How much trouble is she going to be in?" "I wonder why you think Nancy's going to hate you?," I asked Debra. "I told on her. If you would have known I wouldn't of had to squeal on her," said Debra. "Yeah, you really put Debra and well all of us in a bad position, I mean it's not your fault that you didn't see it, but really, what a burden for the rest of us," said Tina. "Do others feel similarly," I asked. "Sort of," said Clare, "But I also keep thinking you truly had no idea and then I started feeling bad for you–just like I do now. You have all this heat on you." "I feel like my typical asshole self," said Mona. "I wanted to say something so bad. From the start I wanted to say, **cut it out Nancy**. What are you doing? How can you do that in front of us, but instead I was my usual sheepish, can't speak up, self." "I'm not mad at Nancy or you. I'm mad at me." "That's just how I feel," said Denise, "I wanted to yell **Stop it Nancy** but the words would not come out." "It's just like Mona said." "For me I wasn't sure what the rules were," said Julie. "I didn't know whether or not there was some kind of patient code whereby we all stick together. I wanted to say something but I didn't want to create any turmoil with the rest of the girls. I gotta live here for at least another week." "What about you Liz," I asked. "I don't know. I just checked out when the whole thing was going on. Who cares right? Let's just move on to a new scene." "I don't know about that Liz–I think we need to stick with this one." I responded.

This case scenario in which the therapist did not see the self-destructive behavior imposed by one of the group members fueled the group with themes that included lack of the protector's (therapist) awareness, feelings of aloneness during frightening times, feelings of need to take care of the perceived weak therapist, not being able to assert oneself, feelings of disloyalty, feelings of ambivalence around the disclosure of secrets, wishes to be taken care of, feelings of fear, anger, and disappointment, and the use of disassociation. These themes spilled over into my individual work with each of these clients.

Powerful transferences evoked via the disability. For example, sometimes clients from the group enacted scenes from childhood in which their mothers were unaware of an incestual experience. Other times, they worked through feelings of self-blame they had carried for years because they did not speak up. Other clients discussed the disappointment they experienced in their parents and compared it to the disappointment they felt from me that day. For others, it was their anger that resurfaced and for still others feelings of fear and not being safe. In Liz's case, we were able to explore her well-developed yet defeating defense of disassociation. Still others developed transferences in which I was cast into their weak, vulnerable caretaker. When however, I was able to sustain hearing their thoughts, feelings, unconventional activity, and secrets, they began to think that perhaps too their caregivers, mainly mothers, could also survive their true selves. I continued to work with many of these young girls for the next six months to the next six years. Throughout the duration, therapeutic material continued to be generated from this group.

In the years that followed, Debra and I had developed a metaphoric language. After explaining something to me in session, she would often ask, do you understand or are you still in the dark? Sometimes I would tell her I was still lurking in the dark, and suggest she give me more information to shed some light. I would advise her to be loud and clear just like she was that day in the group. We would laugh together as we moved towards a brighter life.

There is very little literature to draw from which addresses the pros and cons of working with therapists with disabilities let along therapists who have no or low vision. In one of two articles that currently exist, Ceconi and Urdange (1994) examine the limitations, compensatory issues, and unexpected opportunities that can emerge from working with a social worker who is blind. While providing good eye contact is an important aspect of creating a positive therapeutic relationship (Schaefor, Horejsk, & Horejsi (2000), Ceconi and Urdange have found that "being looked at" can evoke uncomfortable feelings for others especially those experiencing an overwhelming sense of shame. In some cases, the anonymity that can come from having a social worker who is blind, makes one feel more secure (Ceconi & Urdange, 1994). These social workers are careful to note the profound communication that is transmitted non-verbally, however, they also wonder if the absence of sight can provide a deeper understanding by the clinician. Ceconi and Urdange are careful to remind us that blind therapists are not a homogeneous group. They have become blind at different times, in different ways, and have varying degrees of adaptation all lending to their therapeutic effectiveness.

Theories Regarding the Treatment of Persons with Disabilities

There is little written on psychotherapy with persons who are physically disabled (Grzesiak & Hicok, 1994). Historically physical disability was viewed similarly to mental illness. Spirits and demons were alleged to be the cause of various physical afflictions (Ehrenwald, 1976). Up until the start of the 19th century people with disabilities were seen by faith-healers, shamans, magicians, and exorcists. Most of the physically challenged like the mentally ill were incarcerated or institutionalized in deplorable conditions (Ehrenwald, 1976).

Freud and Disability

Freud never elaborated on the psychology of physical disability as he was more interested in the manifestations of intrapsychic conflict. Infer-ences have been made, however, from illustrations included in his work (Grzesiak & Hicok, 1994). He did however, highlight the experience of loss in the understanding of acquired disabilities and physical illness. Since then many of his contemporaries have drawn upon his Mourning and Melancholia to better understand the intraphysic processes that en-able a person to sustain a significant loss (Grezesiak & Hicok, 1994). Generally, a pure psychoanalytic approach (Psychoanalysis) is not a preferred treatment intervention for persons with disabilities as the physical impairment is typically not a result of intraphysic conflict (Gresiak & Hicok, 1994).

Ego Psychology

The school of ego psychology stemmed from Freud's structural model (id, ego, super-ego), and was further developed by his daughter Anna and her contemporaries including Heinz Hamman, Ernst Kris, Alfred Lowenstein, David Rapaport, and Erik Erikson (Goldstein, 1995). Ego psychology views disabilities as traumatic experiences, especially acquired disabilities and maintains a focus on ego functions and ego defenses (Grzesiak & Hicok, 1944). The most common used defenses in response to physical disability are denial, repression, projection, reaction formation, and regression (Cubbage & Thomas, 1989). Anna Freud (1952) is careful to remind us that the age of which the illness or disability emerges has a significant impact on one's developing ego, identity, and body image.

While defenses were central to the ego in Freud's theory, Heinz Hartman initially introduced the autonomous functions of the ego which include such operations as judgment, reality testing, throught processes, and mother activity. According to Goldstein (1995) ego functions are the fundamental mechanisms by which the individual adapts to the external world. Hartman (1939) posited that individuals are born "preadapted" to an "average expectable environment." While Hartman's contributions are seminal to the general understanding of the ego and its functions, Fraiberg's (1970) study of the development of blind babies alerts us that babies born blind do not embark upon an average expectable environment as they enter this world. Fraiberg suggests that "while a mother with a high degree of adaptation and mother love will predictably respond favorably to her infant's needs, that same mother can be challenged by an infant born blind" (p. 120). These observations suggest that the social worker who is helping his/her client with a disability through the lens of ego psychology, may want to access not only the adaptive functioning and ego strengths of the client, but other family members as well particularly when working with children. Cohen (2005) further suggests that the family's financial resources, time, flexibility of family roles as well as the family's capacity to deal with stress be considered during the client's assessment as these factors may have great bearing on the client's future coping and adaptation, as well.

Object Relations Theory

While object relations theory is rooted in some general Freudian beliefs, it moves away from the focus on psychic energy, adaptive functioning (ego psychology), and into a more relational sphere of understanding human development. Object relations theory highlights the interactions individuals have with significant others in their lives, the internalizations of these interactions, and the future role these experiences have in one's psychological development (Melano-Flanagan, 1996). Historically, two distinct schools of object relations theory emerged; the British School and the American School. Leading contributors of the British School included Melanie Klein, W. R. D. Fairbairn, Harry Guntrip, John Bowlby, and D. W. Winicott. The American School included such clinical scholars as Otto Kernberg, Margaret Mahler, and James Masterson (Melano-Flanagan, 1996). This following discussion will borrow concepts from Winicott's conception of object relations theory to understand disabilities. I will focus on two specific Winicottian concepts; the *holding environment* and the development of the *true self.*

When social workers inform their therapeutic approach through an object relations framework, they will often refer to providing a stable holding environment for their clients in order that the client can freely explore their inner and outer worlds. In other words, the social worker is providing a safe and secure physical and mental space for their clients to take risks, experience feelings, identify conflicts, and discover themselves. Clients who most easily integrate into their new holding environment are people who have generally internalized a sense of safety and security from past holding environments; the most influential being the one they were born into.

Babies initially develop a sense of being "held" in the most literal way. While it is important for all babies to have tactile stimulation from their caregivers throughout infancy, it is crucial to the healthy psychological development of children born blind (Fraiberg, 1970). As babies mature, they can continue to develop a sense of psychological security from watching their caregivers, looking at the familiar surroundings of their environments, and/or exchanging a smile with a parent or significant other from across the room. Blind babies are excluded from receiving all visual stimuli which we know is an effective interchange and leads to healthy objective relations in the future. In Fraiberg's (1970) study on blind infants, she concluded that the lack of ongoing tactile stimulation in some cases lead to autistic behaviors in blind children. She observed that some parents did not engage in much physical contact with their children, nor did they provide much auditory stimulation, although they spent much time in the presence of their children. As a result, Fraiberg suspects that the sighted siblings of these blind children did not develop autistic behaviors because they were able to compensate for the lack of physical closeness with their parents through other means of connection, mainly visual observations. In this same study, Fraiberg highlighted the healthy sense of self one blind baby "Robbie" had developed despite his mother's pathology. In this case Robbie's obese mother literally held him all the time. While Fraiberg notes that this probably would have resulted in repercussions for sighted-children who would have needed more freedom to explore, it was essential to Robbie's development as he was in a different developmental stage from his sighted cohorts. It is important to note that the time frame for achieving expectable biological psychological, social, and cognitive milestones of development vary for children with physical disabilities (Cohen, 2005). In addition children with physical disabilities often require very different interactional patterns with their caregivers in order to develop a healthy sense of self.

Winicott believed that at the core of personality was one's *true self* which can only be achieved through a genuine attachment to another (Winicott, 1960). This true self develops through the mutual trust that is established between the caregiver and child which allows both individuals to express their uniqueness, individuality and difference (Melano-Flangan, 1996). There are countless stories from clients that describe a lifetime in which they have had to deny or suppress their own feelings, experiences, wishes, and sometimes the disability itself in order to protect a parent from feelings of guilt, shame, inadequacy, etc., in response to having a child with a disability. Helton (1999), on the other hand, offers an empowering case example of a blind mother and her two blind sons with special needs who could "see" far beyond what most healthcare professionals could. In this narrative, the social worker describes a mother who fosters the true self of her sons through her full attention, attunement, and unconditional acceptance of their limitations. Hetton (1999) writes, "She had a soothing style of speaking with the boys when they had behavioral outbursts or began to self-stimulate" (p. 57).

Rational Emotive Behavioral Therapy (REBT)

REBT is a brief treatment model that draws upon cognitive ideas, behavioral concepts, humanistic principles and constructivist ideology (Ellis, 2001), although some critics believe that Ellis is a bit far-reaching (Kottler, 2002). I have included a discussion of REBT because its' founder Albert Ellis has identified himself as having multiple disabilities and challenges including easily tired eyes, hearing loss, renal glycosuria and diabetes. He goes on to suggest that all of these issues present themselves in the therapy room and often he needs to acknowledge his unconventional behavior with his clients. For example, he may need to close his eyes during a therapy session or eat a small meal in the presence of a client to keep his blood sugar level in a stable state (Ellis, 1997).

According to REBT, individuals posses a number of irrational beliefs that can significantly affect their behavior and ultimately lead to many life compromises including pathological states such as depression, substance abuse, and anxiety disorders. Ellis identifies the two primary contributors to human neurosis as having a low frustration tolerance and possessing self-denigrating thoughts. Ellis espouses that people with disabilities are at high risk for experiencing both frustration and self-denigrating thoughts because society is not particularly accommodating and most people have much bias towards the abilities of those with disabilities. While Ellis's assessment is empathic, his cure seems a bit harsh. He recommends that people with disabilities like himself quit whining. To his benefit he further elaborates that people employ REBT, which teaches one to evaluate their thoughts, feelings, and actions rather than themselves (Ellis, 2001). Ellis (1997) sees himself as a role model to his clients with disabilities and he believes that he demonstrates courage and self-acceptance.

While REBT can be a very effective therapy, it seems that disabilities are quite complicated and this model seems to have a tendency to simplify the implications of having a disability. Anecdotal evidence from several clients suggest that if they could so easily change their way of thinking about their disabilities, they would do it, but "it's not that simple." Ellis on the other hand, reports great success with using REBT with clients with disabilities (Ellis, 1997).

The Ecological Perspective

The Ecological Perspective is the hallmark model of generalist social work practice. It takes into account the person (family, group, community, and organization) in the context of his/her immediate environment and larger environment as well. The ecological model provides a broader conceptualization of disability. It recognizes the history of discrimination against people with disabilities, the structural impact of government policies, cultural assumptions about the capabilities of people with disabilities, and the impact of the disability on the individual, his/her family and the biological and psychological aspects that are part of the disorder (Morales & Shaefor, 2001). Today, it is also important to understand the spiritual significance or religious convictions a disability might evoke. All of these factors can profoundly impact the problems and solutions of the client's issues related to his/her disability. As Cohen (2005) states the application of an ecological perspective to social work assessment and practice is critical to the understanding of disabilities through the generations.

Given the breadth and depth the ecological model promotes, the social worker may assume a range of roles at different times depending on the immediate needs of the client. For example, a client may be working with a social worker to deal with the experience or loss following an acquired disability, however, the client's need for alternative transportation to the next appointment may require that the social worker temporarily depart from the role of counselor and function in the role of broker in order that a successful means of transportation is identified, and the necessary referral made. That some social workers may soon find himself/herself at a meeting with the client and his/her boss advocating for the client's return to work.

Within the framework of the ecological model, social workers can help persons with disabilities on a micro, mezzo, and macro level. Social workers have taken a leading role in providing services to persons with disabilities, although the infusion of disability content within the social work curriculum seems to lag behind other issues of diversity. While there has been remarkable advances in terms of public policy and resources available to persons with disabilities, we have far to go. The professional commitment of social workers to this cause lends great promise, to advancing the quality of life for all individuals with disabilities.

REFERENCES

Asch, A., & Rousso, H. (1985). Therapists with disabilities: Theoretical and clinical issues. *Psychiatry, 48*, 1-12.

Beck, R. (1991). The hearing-impaired psychotherapist: Implications for process and practice. *Clinical Social Work Journal 19*(4), 417-426.

Ceconi, B., & Urdang, E. (1994). Sight or insight: Child therapy with a blind clinician. *Clinical Social Work Journal, 22*(2), 179-192.

Cubbage, M., & Thomas, K. (1989). Freud and disability. *Rehabilitation Psychology, 34*, 161-173.

Diller, J. (1999). *Cultural diversity: A primer for the human services.* Belmont, CA: Wadsworth Publishing Company.

Ehrenwald, J. (1976). *A history of psychotherapy.* New York: Jason Aronson.

Ellis, A. (1997). Using rational emotive behavioral therapy techniques to cope with disability. *Professional Psychology: Research and Practice, 28*(1), 17-22.

Ellis, A. (2001). *Overcoming destructive beliefs, feelings, and behaviors: New directions for rational emotive behavior therapy.* New York: Prometheus.

Fraiberg, S. (1970). The muse in the kitchen: A case study in clinical research. *Smith College Studies in Social Work, XL*(2), 101-134.

Freud, A. (1952). The role of bodily illness in the mental life of children. *Psychoanalytic Study of the Child, VII* (pp. 430-453). New York: International Universities Press.

Germain, C., & Gitterman, A. (1996). *The life model of social work practice.* New York: Columbia University Press.

Goldstein, E. (1995). *Ego psychology and social work practice.* New York: The Free Press.

Grzesiak, R., & Hicok, D. (1994). A brief history of psychotherapy and physical disability. *American Journal of Psychotherapy, 48*(2), 240-251.

Harsh, M. (1993). Women who are visually impaired or blind as psychotherapy clients: A personal and professional perspective. *No men and therapy, 14*(3/4), 55-64.

Hartman, H. (1939). *Ego psychology and the problem of adaptation.* New York: International Universities Press.

Helton, L. (1999). From my view everything is clear: Building on family strengths. *Reflections*, (Fall), 53-63.

Hyman, H. L. (2003). Out of sight: A personal journey through ten months of blindness. *Generations.* EBSCO Publishing, 108-110.

Kohut, H. (1977). *Restoration of the self.* New York: International Universities Press.

Kottler, J. (2002). *Theories in counseling and therapy: An experiential approach.* Boston: Allyn and Bacon.

Melano-Flanagan, L. (1996). Object relations theory. In J. Berzoff, L. Melano-Flanagan, & P. Hertz (Eds.), *Inside out and outside in: Psychodynamic clinical theory and practice in contemporary multicultural contexts* (pp. 128-171). Northvale, NJ: Jason Aronson.

Morales, A. & Sheafor, B. (2001). *Social work: A profession of many faces.* Boston: Allyn and Bacon.

Pillari, V. (2002). *Social work practice: Theories and skills.* Boston: Allyn and Bacon.

Schamess, G. (1996). Ego psychology. In J. Berzoff, L. Melano Flanagan, & P. Hertz (Eds.), *Inside out and outside in: Psychodynamic clinical theory and practice in contemporary multicultural contexts* (pp. 67-101). Northvale, NJ: Jason Aronson, Inc.

Schulman, L. (1999). *The skill of helping individuals, groups, families, and communities* (4th ed.). Itasca, IL: E. E. Peacock.

Sheafor, B., Horejsi, C., & Horejsi, G. (2000). *Techniques and guidelines for social work practice* (5th ed.). Boston: Allyn and Bacon.

Tams, S. F. (1998). Comparing the self-concept of persons with and without physical disabilities. *Journal of Psychology, 132*(1), 78-87.

Vision Connections (2004). http.www.visionconnections.org.

Wahl, H. W., Schilling, O., Oswald, F., & Heyl, V. (1999). Psychosocial consequences of age-related visual impairment: Comparison with mobility-impaired older adults and long-term outcome. *Journal of Gerontology Psychological Sciences, 54B*(5), 304-316.

Winicott, D. W. (1960). *Ego distortion in terms of true and false self.* London: Hogarth.

Yorke, C. (1980). Some comments on the psychoanalytic treatment of patients with physical disabilities. *International Journal of Psycho-Analysis, 161,* 187-193.

doi:10.1300/J198v06n01_09

Disability and Spirituality
in Social Work Practice

Jane Hurst

SUMMARY. In working with social work clients, issues of religion and spirituality are sure to arise. Religious views on disability can have both positive and negative effects on the individual. In our increasingly pluralistic society, these issues must be approached with sensitivity and patience since it is common to work with adherents of minority or non-traditional religious groups or groups whose values conflict with the social work profession. The purpose of this article is to enhance and develop sensitivity to diverse religious views in order to respect the values and life beliefs of the client while enhancing the development of adaptive religious and spiritual views. doi:10.1300/J198v06n01_10 *[Article copies available for a fee from The Haworth Document Delivery Service: 1-800-HAWORTH. E-mail address: <docdelivery@haworthpress.com> Website: <http://www.HaworthPress.com> © 2007 by The Haworth Press, Inc. All rights reserved.]*

KEYWORDS. Spirituality, religion, suffering, acceptance, inclusion, compassion, non-violence

---

Jane Hurst, PhD, is Chair, Department of Philosophy & Religion, Gallaudet University, Hall Memorial Building, Room S-134, 800 Florida Avenue NE, Washington, DC 20002 (E-mail: Jane.Hurst@gallaudet.edu).

[Haworth co-indexing entry note]: "Disability and Spirituality in Social Work Practice." Hurst, Jane. Co-published simultaneously in *Journal of Social Work in Disability & Rehabilitation* (The Haworth Press, Inc.) Vol. 6, No. 1/2, 2007, pp. 179-194; and: *Disability and Social Work Education: Practice and Policy Issues* (ed: Francis K. O. Yuen, Carol B. Cohen, and Kristine Tower) The Haworth Press, Inc., 2007, pp. 179-194. Single or multiple copies of this article are available for a fee from The Haworth Document Delivery Service [1-800-HAWORTH, 9:00 a.m. - 5:00 p.m. (EST). E-mail address: docdelivery@haworthpress.com].

INTRODUCTION

When working with clients who are experiencing either permanent or temporary disability, issues of spirituality are a key to helping them work through the many issues surrounding such disabilities. There are two perspectives we can take toward disability and spirituality. The first is from the point of view of the client, who may or may not have a spiritual perspective on the experience of disability. This spiritual perspective, in turn, may be either harmful or helpful to the client's life adjustment. In our increasingly pluralistic society, these issues must be approached with sensitivity and patience since it is common to come across adherents of minority or non-traditional religious groups, or adherents of groups with which the social worker is either unfamiliar or does not personally approve.

The second major perspective is from that of the social worker. All of us have emotional responses when confronted with disability, either our own or that of others. Some possible categories of response are romanticization, judgment, fear, denial, and hope. In training, and especially under supervised practice, these responses can be examined and understood by the social worker. Inevitably, one's own spiritual life has an impact on how one understands and works with clients. In the end, a growing awareness of where one stands on spiritual issues helps the social worker to develop empathy for views that are not his or her own, and to help the client develop a constructive, life-affirming attitude that incorporates a spiritual perspective.

Issues of spirituality are among the most sensitive in social work practice. When personal beliefs are held strongly, by either the client or the social worker, the possibility for conflict is equally strong. For example, a client in a fragile personal situation may develop a physical disability, such as lower back pain. If this client is a believer in New Age alternative healing and has a strong commitment to the power of prayer to heal all things, she might refuse a consultation with a doctor, pain-relieving medication, and physical therapy. The social worker, coming from a secular perspective, might find this simply appalling. His or her more rational analysis might find the refusal to seek conventional treatment to be an expression of a self-destructive tendency in the client, or of malingering, or of a kind of closed-mindedness that does not effectively allow problem solving.

The only hope for this kind of stalemate situation is through the personal exploration and growth of both the client and the social worker. The social worker is ethically bound to meet the client where he or she is and work from there. In practice, great care must be taken in any attempt to change a client's religious orientation or belief system. This is where self knowledge is very important, so that one's process with the client does not come from a need to impose one's own views, but from the needs of the client him or herself. This is challenging and difficult territory.

So what is the social worker to do? What is the most effective way to work with clients to integrate possible new perspectives that would enhance their lives and adjustment to disability, while maintaining their personal faith? How can social workers maintain their own religious or spiritual stands while respecting and honoring those who might have a totally different view of these issues? In this essay, we will explore the answers to these questions.

A NOTE ON THE DEFINITIONS
OF RELIGION AND SPIRITUALITY

Just as people have differing religious or spiritual beliefs, they also have strongly held beliefs about the terms *religion* and *spirituality*. Many adherents of what outsiders consider to be religions do not consider their group to be a religion but rather the One True Way. Others have had negative experiences with organized religion, and therefore consider the term itself to be negative and limiting. They prefer the term *spirituality* to refer to their inner spiritual life and relationship with God.

For the purposes of this essay, we will define *religion* as a set of beliefs, values, rituals, and practices that are held by a group of people concerning their relationship with God, or whatever concept they use to refer to that which is beyond physical reality. These religions can be categorized into major and minor groups, and can be researched by nonbelievers who wish to understand them. (See resource list at the end of this article for internet links and recommended books.) Commonly religions refer to authorities, such as religious leaders or sacred scriptures, for guidance on correct religious belief and practice. *Spirituality* is understood as an individual's personal beliefs, values, rituals and practices in relationship to God or the non-material aspects of the self. It does not depend on outside authority, but rather the individual's experience and study. Individuals may study inspirational literature or study with spiritual teachers or directors, but the real action takes place inside the individual, and not in a group of people.

Thus, a person might be a practitioner of a recognizable religion, and worship in a group setting, but also have a personal, well-developed spirituality. Or a person might be religious and not spiritual, or spiritual and not religious, or of course neither religious nor spiritual. All of these options are to be expected in social work practice. The social worker, when confronted with a client who has a strong religious or spiritual perspective, should ideally do some objective questioning to elicit exactly where the client stands on these issues, and some research to provide background to deepen understanding of where the client is coming from, including consulting with religious leaders. In this essay, we will explore some examples of how this might work.

NEGATIVE RELIGIOUS AND SPIRITUAL ATTITUDES TOWARD PEOPLE WITH DISABILITIES

The variety of possible ways to live as a human being is such a vast array of possibility that the mind cannot hold it all at one time. For this reason, most of us assume, perhaps unconsciously, that the way we are living is the standard by which all others are judged and proceed from there. Even when our lives do not conform to some cultural or personal inner standard, we may still have expectations about what life should be. When confronted with disability, these expectations crumble and must be replaced with new paradigms on how life can be lived in a healthy, creative, and constructive way.

Religions have confronted disability in several main ways that are negative in their approach. For the purposes of this discussion we will categorize these as judgmental, as opportunities to demonstrate faith, and as romanticized notions of suffering. Note that all three of these perspectives are not particularly interested in what the disabled person has to say about his or her own experience. They assume the passivity of the person with a disability as an object upon whom the "normal people" gaze with varying attitudes of disapproval, pity, and unrealistic expectation.

For example, in the New Testament Mark 7:32-37 (The New English Bible, 1976), a deaf man is brought to Jesus for healing, which he does with the phrase "*Ephphatha*" (be opened). The disciples are amazed at Jesus' healing ability. "Their astonishment knew no bounds: 'All that he does, he does well,' they said; 'he even makes the deaf hear and the dumb speak'" (The New English Bible, 1976, Mark 7:37). In this story, the focus is Jesus' healing power, not the deaf man. No one stops to ask this man if he wanted to be healed, how he felt about the process, or what thinks of changes this will bring in his life. He is used by the gospel writer to tell a story about Jesus, and not seen as a complete, holistic person himself. Joseph P. Shapiro responds to this sort of attitude in his book *No Pity: People with Disabilities Forging a New Civil Rights Movement* (1993). He urges people who do not live with disabilities to get beyond fear and prejudice and projection and actually ask people with disabilities about their lives. Shapiro says that people with disabilities "insist simply on common respect and the opportunity to build bonds to their communities as fully accepted participants in everyday life" (Shapiro, 1993:332).

The social worker's challenge here is to get past the position of looking at the person who is living with a disability as the "other" and begin to see this person as part of the range of possible ways to live as a human being. If the social worker himself or herself holds some of these negative religious assumptions, this might be a challenge. In addition, people with disabilities may be members of religious groups that hold some attitudes that from an outsider's perspective may look negative and not very constructive to a healthy identity and self-understanding. Here is where the social worker must exercise utmost sensitivity, based on self-awareness of his or her own religious and spiritual perspective and an openness to the perspectives of others.

There are specific social work values that social workers must adhere to, whatever their religious orientation. For example if the Catholic Church says that homosexuality is morally unacceptable and the social worker is Catholic, the social worker is bound by the code of ethics to view homosexual people from a diversity perspective which accepts diverse minority populations. In the case of religion and disability, this understanding is twofold, in that it considers respect for diverse religious views and for diversity among disabled people. To help in this process of understanding, we will now look at these three major ways that religions have viewed disability, first in their negative forms, and then in the next section in their more positive manifestations.

Disability as God's Judgment

Religions have many social functions, the most obvious being a way to keep groups together with explicit rules to govern behavior and shared values and meanings for the group. The easiest way to enforce this kind of group unity is through fear of negative consequences if someone deviates from the religious consensus, i.e., fear of God's judgment.[1] Whether you are a religious person or not, it is clear that when you look at most religious belief systems, people follow certain moral rules because they fear what would happen if they did not. In fact, many people will directly tell you that if you are not a member of their particular faith, you are in danger of "going to hell." There is sometimes an almost superstitious attitude, and it is probably unconscious, that you can ward off negative events by following a straight and narrow spiritual path.

This works perfectly until reality sets in, and bad things happen to good people. And they always do, since sickness and death and disappointment are inevitable facts of life. So how does the religious person respond? The first response is often that these kinds of events are "God's Will," which means that God had a reason for bringing this difficult event at this time in this way to you. Underneath this is an often unstated, and sometimes clearly articulated, assumption that you must have done something wrong to bring this on yourself. If you had only had more faith, or lived a more perfect life, this never would have happened in the first place. In the case of disability, the parents of a child with a disability might blame themselves, or the adult disabled by an accident or illness might search for personal imperfections that might have brought this about. All of these assume that God makes these things happen as some kind of punishment.

Disability as a Lack of Faith

This leads to the second way religions sometimes regard people with disabilities, as opportunities to demonstrate faith by trying to heal them. A student at Gallaudet University, where I have taught Philosophy and Religion for 25 years, once approached me and asked me to comment on something his boss had told him: "If you had more faith you would be able to hear."[2] This is appalling in its judgmental approach and in the way it ties faith in God with observable events in the material world. Over and over again, people with disabilities are approached on the street or taken to Church where the faithful pray over them and ask God for healing.

I do not have a quarrel with the truly good hearted religious folks who want to alleviate the suffering in the world, but when this objectifies the person who is disabled, and assumes they are suffering without asking them, it is clearly unacceptable. In social science terms, in such cases members of religious groups are attempting to heal disabled people as a way of proving that their own religious faith is true. This reinforces their own group membership and identity. What is troubling is that the disabled person is not heard from, and is made into a proof of faith, rather than respected and acknowledged as a complete human being.

THE NOBILITY OF SUFFERING

The third way religions can regard people with disabilities also objectifies them by projecting a romantic idea of the nobility of suffering onto those who struggle with physical and mental challenges. This comes from ideas of suffering in the Bible (Job in the Hebrew Bible who suffers to test his faith, Jesus on the Cross in the New Testament who suffers and dies for the sins of humanity) and from a history of suffering by both Jews and Christians throughout history. The long tradition of martyrdom from Masada, through the early persecuted Christians to the suffering endured by the medieval saints for the sake of holiness carries forth this theme. For example in Isaiah we meet the "suffering servant" through whose suffering the people of Israel will realize atonement. "Yet on himself he bore our sufferings, our torments he endured . . . he was pierced for our transgressions, tortured for our iniquities; the chastisement he bore is health for us and by his scourging we are healed" (The New English Bible, 1976, Isaiah 53:4-5).

If you ask anyone with a chronic condition that causes suffering, it is not an automatically ennobling experience. Pain can be a teacher, yes, but most of the time it is just pain that gets in the way of living your life as fully as possible. Individuals respond to disability in as diverse a number of ways as there are human beings, and to lump these people together as the "noble suffering servant" does them a great disservice.

Here is an opportunity for the social worker to take some time and ask the client about his or her experience of disability, of personal struggle, of life's challenges. The answers might be surprising. For Deaf people, for example, being Deaf per se is not a disability, but the fact that so much of the world does not use sign language and therefore is not accessible in terms of communication is a considerable challenge in life. Hard of hearing people who do not use sign and are not culturally deaf might have a different view, ranging from "so what?" to pride in meeting the challenge of functioning in a world that is so oriented toward the hearing. Someone in a serious car accident who miraculously lives through it, though now uses a wheel chair for mobility, might be so happy to be alive that the "disability" is hardly an issue. Christopher Reeve was an example of the courageous, self-accepting disabled person who was also focused on personal healing. Such disability might cause much more disabling personal adjustment problems for an athlete sidelined by injury in his or her prime, especially if that person had never previously engaged in much self-reflection.

The best description of negative religious attitudes toward people with disabilities that I have found is Rev. Nancy Lane's article "Victim Theology" (Lane, 2001). In it she describes and analyzes her experience as a minister, a person living with cerebral palsy, and as a woman of faith. In this essay, she examines what she calls "victim theology" and the ways that it uses biblical teachings to "judge, dismiss, and disempower us, usually shutting us out of the religious community" (Lane, 2001, 1). This article is highly recommended for anyone working with clients who have a strong faith perspective, whether disabled or not. Lane makes an impassioned statement calling for inclusion on a deep level.

> Those of us who live with disability, who have plumbed the depths of our experiences of grace and limitation, of loss and survival, of grief and joy, of oppression and crying out, have much to bring to the theology and spirituality of seeking, finding and knowing God. It is simply a matter of acceptance and inclusion, of being welcomed into the community, where our stories and experiences are heard and received as part of the ongoing history of God in the world. (Lane, 2001, 13)

Rev. Lane has found a way to personally get past the negative attitude in "victim theology" and maintain her faith. The kinds of more positive attitudes that might encourage this possibility are in the next section.

POSITIVE RELIGIOUS AND SPIRITUAL ATTITUDES TOWARD PEOPLE WITH DISABILITIES

Disability as the Unfolding of God's Plan

For people of faith, the idea that God has a plan for each life is often a strongly held personal belief. All human beings suffer, so that the suffering each person undergoes is personally designed to help that person grow and develop. Rather than being a punishment, experiencing setbacks whether temporary or permanent are opportunities for learning and maturing and deepening one's faith. Some folks experience the easy, "gut" course in life, while others are on the accelerated Honors track. There is no judgment here, just taking in stride whatever life produces as evidence of God's love and guidance. It is important to note that what may appear to be "punishment" from God is not so in this perspective, but rather a gift which can be treasured and used as a path to greater faith and the experience of love in the world.

For the social worker working with a client who has a strong faith position, this view of God's plan for people's lives is much more healthy than the judgmental, guilt producing, and integrity denying approach in the previous section. If you are comfortable, you can work with a client in his or her own faith tradition to try to find examples of this perspective. If you are not comfortable, it might be helpful to have a list of clergy who can serve as resources for referring your clients who want to have this religious perspective become part of their healing process. Your local area may have a directory of religious groups and their leaders, and you might need to do some field work to find clergy who have a positive perspective on disability. One warning about this referral process is that it must be done only with the client's wholehearted approval, and it obviously must not be done as a way to push one's own religious beliefs on the client. In fact, boundaries might be better maintained if the social worker who has a church home refers the client to a pastor other than his or her own.

Disability as an Opportunity for Strengthening Faith

Faith is easy when things are going well. When confronted with obstacles, maintaining faith is a challenge. Real faith is a response to an ongoing interaction with life from the perspective of a relationship with God. It is active, not passive, and as such is not based on "what God has done for me" or "what I believe in" in an external sense. Faith is an inward quality that gains its strength from life's vicissitudes. Because it is so difficult to maintain, faith is precious.

The social worker who engages with a client who expresses a religious faith can work with the client to help him or her develop this more sophisticated understanding of faith. Practically speaking, it may require a lot of work to get through anger and depression to get to this position. Denial of these feelings is also possible, so the social worker must be aware of any attempt to gloss over negative feelings in a jump to acceptance. This process is hard work.

Ideally, the question "Why did God do this to me?" which arises from despair and which presupposes a victim consciousness, can be transformed into "How can this experience allow me to deepen and strengthen my faith and my relationship with God." This is not an easy task, but if it were easy it would not be such a precious process. And it is an empowering process which takes the victim mentality and changes it to the mentality of a triumphant survivor. Social workers would need to understand the client's anger, facilitate the grief process and then focus on the religious aspects in order to facilitate this empowerment process.

Disability and Suffering as a Way to Compassion

His Holiness the Dalai Lama of Tibet writes extensively about the spiritual sickness he sees in the West, a sickness of mind and heart that leads us to believe we are separate from each other, that we are in competition with each other, and that we give only so that we can get. His solution for this problem of the modern world is the development of Compassion in which we experience the pain and joy of others from the depth of our own hearts. When we do so, we create a world of unity, co-operation and generosity. We surrender our passivity in the face of cultural values that do not serve us and become empowered as loving, caring, compassionate human beings.

For a person with a disability this is an especially important endeavor because mainstream culture so consistently marginalizes and disregards the interests and contributions of disabled people. The feeling of imposed passivity is infuriating and insulting. Are we not all equal as human beings, with the same capacities for interaction with our lives? It is fear of one another that can block this understanding, and to people who have not experienced disability, the physical limitations of others can be terrifying, and thus lead the able-bodied to dismiss the disabled person as unimportant as a way of handling this projected fear.

The disabled person has a great opportunity to develop compassion in this situation. The fear that keeps us all from becoming fully human is there in all of us. Because the disabled person has more cause to confront that fear when working toward a healthy stance toward his or her physical or mental limitations, he or she can develop more awareness of the way fear limits our lives. I don't mean this as an automatic understanding bestowed upon any person with a disability, but rather as the hard fought stance of the person who has faced down fear and limitation and emerged to live life with creativity and joy.

For the disabled person compassion is the healthy response to the fear and projections and judgments of others. It also might be mixed with a fair dose of anger and frustration and all the other possible emotions that arise in difficult situations. But compassion is empowering, for it meets other human beings on a totally equal spiritual footing. This is what Mahatma Gandhi pointed to when he talked about *satyagraha*, the soul force present in every human being in equal measure no matter what one's age or race or religion or physical condition. This powerful force is there in all of us, said Gandhi, and is the energy behind our endeavors on behalf of one another. It is the energy behind his teachings of non-violent political and social action.

Compassion, based on the understanding of all of us as equal in our amount of soul force and in our capacity to love one another, is one of the qualities that makes a great social worker rather than a merely good one. As differentiated from pity, which desires to help others as a way to make oneself feel good, compassion is a shared celebration of connection with others. In such a situation, we each use our skills to help one another, but it is by no means obvious who is helping who.

Compassion is not something that can be "believed in" or taught. As such, compassion falls more into the category of spirituality rather than religion. Compassion is something that grows out of experiencing life. When faced with fear and an urge to contract and separate, compassion goes the opposite direction and chooses love and expansion and connection. As we consider the ways of working with spirituality in a therapeutic setting, we can see how mutual compassion creates a healthy process.

Many clients coming into a healing environment have not have not been understood or had an empathic connection (Kohut) so necessary for a sense of self and well being. When social workers make an empathic, compassionate connection with their clients, they have the capacity to bring about profound healing.

SPIRITUALITY FOR CLIENTS AND SOCIAL WORKERS

Much of this essay thus far has looked at religious views that might possibly be encountered in the client-social worker relationship. This is important, because these are the most common religious attitudes in our culture, and these will be the attitudes that both client and social worker will have to deal with in one way or another. As a social worker, it is very important to do a rigorous program of self-analysis so that you know where you stand on religious and spiritual issues. Once this has been done, you have a place to work from to understand and support the religious and spiritual views of others.

This need to know where one stands also applies to spirituality, one's personal beliefs, values, rituals and practices in relationship to God or the non-material aspects of the self. These would not necessarily be arrived at through experience in a group or from transmission from an authority figure. Rather, they are the individual's expression of the things usually categorized as religious that have gone through a process of study, reflection, and prayer to be internalized by that individual.

An individual social worker may or may not have an interest in developing a personal spirituality. Whether or not you wish to do so is a question you must ask yourself. If not, then you need to work to develop a way to work with clients who are personally interested in this. Again, a referral list is invaluable for getting clients to spiritual groups or teachers or literature that will be helpful to them. If you are personally interested in the spiritual quest, you will have an easier time working with clients who share that interest if you are careful to maintain good boundaries. The key is to remember that you are working for the client's own good and not to convince them of the correctness of your own beliefs and practices.

Accessibility is a potential obstacle can arise when directing clients to spiritual, or for that matter religious, groups. Although the ADA is a wonderful law in terms of employment and housing practices, it does have exemptions for such non-profit groups as religious organizations. The good news is that many churches, synagogues, and other religious groups wish to be inclusive and do their best to ensure such things as wheelchair accessibility. More and more places of worship are accessible.

An exception is sign language interpreting for deaf and hard-of-hearing people. Because it is so expensive, and therefore a real financial challenge to groups operating on a limited budget, many religious and spiritual groups depend on volunteer interpreters. This can be great if the interpreter is great, but also it can be dreadful if the interpreter, though a volunteer and free, cannot be understood by the deaf audience or worse, misinterprets what is being said during the religious service. Sign-language interpretation is more common in mainstream and/or evangelical churches than it is in smaller, unconventional spiritual groups, primarily because they have so few financial resources to hire interpreters. Here again a good list of groups that do have people who can interpret is an invaluable tool.[3] Another possible obstacle to a positive, well-integrated personal spirituality is the tendency of some people to accept as authoritative spiritual teachings that are trivial, fear-producing, and even destructive. As is the case with religion, in spirituality there both constructive and destructive forms. It is a special challenge not to be judgmental about groups or beliefs one personally finds ridiculous or worse, unhealthy for the person's life adjustment. At this point, it is best to not directly challenge a group's truth claims, which might produce a defensive reaction, but to adopt a problem solving stance that encourages the client to work through issues him or herself. Most people exploring spirituality try out many different groups before settling on one that fits their spiritual and social needs. Members enter and leave groups all the time, and patience may be required to wait out a client's commitment to something that the social worker judges to be not very helpful. In the end, the client may leave the group or the social worker may come to see its virtues. In any case, open minded listening and support will see you through.

Despite these possible drawbacks, in conclusion we want to emphasize that the spiritual quest is one worth pursuing. Beneath the dross of "victim theology" and limiting religious beliefs there is spiritual gold to be unearthed. Whether as a member of a religious group or as an individual with a rich inner spiritual life, or perhaps as both, both social workers and their clients can find great sources of strength and guidance in the spiritual quest. As it turns out, this sort of quest is most useful in times of difficulty, and this certainly applies to a person with a disability struggling to deal with an often uncaring and judgmental world.

Let me make it clear that we are not marginalizing the person with a disability, but rather expanding the circle of humanity to be sure that all are included in it. When we understand that every human being suffers and must find inspiration and personal meaning from that suffering, we don't need to categorize ourselves as able-bodied or disabled. We are all variations on a theme of being human. It has been said that we are "spiritual beings having a human experience." In this understanding despite our differences, whether they be physical, mental, emotional, cultural, racial, ethnic, or religious, we are all One. To acknowledge that oneness with another human being is deeply spiritual, and it is a great gift that the spiritually inclined social worker has to offer.

CASE STUDY FOR CONSIDERATION AND DISCUSSION

Helen is a 25-year-old woman with severe arthritis in her hands. She finds herself unable to write for long periods of time, and therefore has been challenged both in school, where test-taking is a challenge, and on the job where using a computer keyboard is a requirement. Her religious faith is a strong one, and she attends services at her evangelical church every Sunday, and Bible study during the week. She considers herself to be a sinner and her arthritis is God's Will that she suffer and pay for her sins. At one point, a friend takes her to a hands-on New Age healer and she receives considerable relief from pain and experiences increased mobility. When Helen tells her pastor about it, he tells her that anyone not healing in the name of Jesus Christ is working for the devil and must be rejected. Helen does not go back to the healer and her symptoms eventually return.

Helen is referred to a social worker because her arthritis has affected her ability to work. The social worker is shocked by Helen's presentation of her own self-understanding. She is herself not a very religious or spiritual person, and the idea that someone would needlessly suffer because of faith is hard to understand. Furthermore, Helen's inability to work is causing her major life stress and difficulty. That Helen would have turned down healing help because it did not come from her church is incomprehensible to the social worker, even though she doesn't particularly believe in faith healing in the first place.

The social worker has a couple of options here. One is to work with Helen to help her come to an understanding of her suffering that allows some healing to be accepted. Helen has taken a part of Christianity and fixated on it. There is a great deal more to the religion than punishment for sin, and in fact Jesus himself performs several miracles of healing. Helen can come to accept healing as part of God's plan, and not reject any attempt to help her. Here problem solving via cognitive therapy would be a useful approach.

Another option for the social worker is to refer Helen to a spiritual counselor in a church close in theology to Helen's own. If Helen accepts only the authority of her religious tradition, finding a faith-based counselor or social worker is ideal. This counselor would be expected to have the skills to help Helen come to a more nuanced understanding of her faith, and to help her be open to healing, whether from traditional or non-traditional medicine.

Whichever path is taken, it is key that the social worker maintain a neutral stance with the client, since any criticism of Helen's faith will be rejected and will lead to a breakdown of trust. Focusing on Helen's own cognitive structure and problem solving process will be much more constructive in the long run.

RESOURCES ON RELIGION AND SPIRITUALITY

Some books to get you started:

Ellwood, R., & McGraw, B. A. (2002). *Many peoples, many faiths: Women and men in the world religions*, (7th ed.). Upper Saddle River, NJ: Prentice-Hall.

Fisher, M. P. (2002). *Living religions*, (5th ed.). Upper Saddle River, NJ: Prentice Hall.

Mulloy, M. (2005). *Experiencing the world's religions: Tradition, challenge, and change,* (3rd ed.). New York: McGraw-Hill.

Smith, H. (1991). *The world's religions: Our great wisdom traditions.* San Francisco: Harper.

There are some excellent online resources on religion and spirituality. Here are a few of them that can guide your search.

http://www.throughtheroof.org An interesting site from Great Britain which has a good discussion of how to make churches accessible to people with a wide range of disabilities.

http://www.fas.harvard.edu/~pluralsm/ The Pluralism Project at Harvard University is an objective, reliable online resource with an excellent list of links, including a state by state list of religious organizations.

http://www.beliefnet.com Search under *Disability* for some disability specific articles, or explore very clear and neutral information on a variety of religious faiths. See also the *Illness and recovery* section.

http://www.religioustolerance.org Another very fair site with a wealth of links and topics, including the interfaith movement.

Lane, Rev. Nancy. *Resource Packet on Disability, Spirituality, and Healing* Syracuse, NY: Center on Human Policy, Syracuse University, 1999. Available online at the Syracuse Center on Human Policy. Search "Rev. Nancy Lane" to find a current link. A wealth of information, easily available. Lane has a wise perspective that is deeply spiritual. Highly recommended.

The National Council of Churches, representing 36 denominations, has a committee on Disabilities, with a report to be found at *http://www.ncccusa.org/nmu/mce/dis/.*

The National Organization on Disability has a Religion and Disability Program. For more information go to *www.nod.org* and click on *Religious Participation*. This group has an *Accessible Congregations Campaign* with a state by state listing of accessible churches.

Two excellent sources of information for social workers are *Journal of Religion, Disability & Health* . . . bridging clinical practice and spiritual support and *Journal of Religion and Spirituality in Social Work*, both available from *http://www.haworthpress.com.*

NOTES

1. For purposes of this essay, I will be primarily discussing the Judeo-Christian perspective, which also shares a great deal with the Islamic perspective. For those whose clients adhere to other faiths, or variations of Christianity, Judaism, or Islam, it is helpful to conduct research on these groups through such websites as *www.belief.net.com*. See Resources on Religion and Spirituality for other options.

2. Because he wanted to keep the job, my student did not respond to this aggressive statement, but did find a another job a few months later.

3. Many communities maintain such lists online. For example the Gallaudet University Office of Campus Ministries has a list of Deaf accessible churches in the D.C. area at *http://sa.gallaudet.edu* (Click on Campus Ministries, then Other Links).

REFERENCES

Abrams, J. Z. (1998). *Judaism and disability: Portrayals in ancient texts from the Tanach through the Bavli.* Washington, D.C.: Gallaudet University Press.

Alston, P., & Vash, C. (Eds.). (2001). Special issue on spirituality and disability, *Journal of Rehabilitation*, Jan-March. Available at *www.looksmart.com* or *www.findarticles.com.*

Eiseland, N. (1994). *The disabled God: Toward a liberatory theology of disability.* Nashville: Abingdon Press.

Eiseland, N., & Saliers, D. E. (1998). *Human disability and the service of God: Reassessing religious practice.* Nashville: Abingdon Press.

Hurst, J. (1995). Disability from the point of view of religion and spirituality, *Disability Studies Quarterly*, Summer.

Lane, N. (1999). *Resource packet on disability, spirituality, and healing.* Syracuse, NY: Center on Human Policy, Syracuse University.

Lane, N. (2001). Victim theology. *Journal of Rehabilitation.* Jan-March. Alexandria, VA: National Rehabilitation Association.

New English Bible with the Apocrypha (The): Oxford study edition (1976). S. Sandmel, M. J. Suggs, & A. J. Tkacik (Eds.). New York: Oxford University Press.

Shapiro, J. P. (1993). *No pity: People with disabilities forging a new Civil Rights movement.* New York: Random House.

Webb-Mitchell, B. (1994). *Unexpected guests at God's banquet: Welcoming people with disabilities into the church.* New York: Crossroad Publishing Co.

doi:10.1300/J198v06n01_10

The Implications of Disability Protests
for Social Work Practice

Sharon N. Barnartt

SUMMARY. This article examines the demands which have been made in the over 800 US protests this author has analyzed. Some demands are cross-disability, meaning they could apply to people with all types of impairments; these include demands for rights and accessibility in all domains. Other demands are disability-specific: they apply to people with specific types of impairments, ranging from mobility impairments to developmental disabilities. Many demands have been related to services, which can be either cross-disability or disability-specific. The paper examines the implications of these demands for social work practice. These include that disability be de-stigmatized by practitioners, that people with disabilities have choices, that they have control over their services, and that all aspects of social work practice be accessible to people with any type of disability. doi:10.1300/J198v06n01_11 *[Article copies available for a fee from The Haworth Document Delivery Service: 1-800-HAWORTH. E-mail address: <docdelivery@haworthpress.com> Website: <http://www.HaworthPress.com> © 2007 by The Haworth Press, Inc. All rights reserved.]*

Sharon N. Barnartt, PhD, is Professor, Department of Sociology, Gallaudet University, 800 Florida Avenue NE, Washington, DC 20002 (E-mail: *sharon.barnartt@gallaudet.edu*).

[Haworth co-indexing entry note]: "The Implications of Disability Protests for Social Work Practice." Barnartt, Sharon N. Co-published simultaneously in *Journal of Social Work in Disability & Rehabilitation* (The Haworth Press, Inc.) Vol. 6, No. 1/2, 2007, pp. 195-215; and: *Disability and Social Work Education: Practice and Policy Issues* (ed: Francis K. O. Yuen, Carol B. Cohen, and Kristine Tower) The Haworth Press, Inc., 2007, pp. 195-215. Single or multiple copies of this article are available for a fee from The Haworth Document Delivery Service [1-800-HAWORTH, 9:00 a.m. - 5:00 p.m. (EST). E-mail address: docdelivery@haworthpress.com].

doi:10.1300/J198v06n01_11

KEYWORDS. Disability rights, disability activism, social movements, protests

INTRODUCTION

There have been a large number of protests about disability issues since 1970.[1] By this author's count there have been at least 800 in the US.[2] These protests have made a large number of demands. Some can be classified as either 'disability rights' nor as 'independent living' (Pfeiffer, 1988). But those are only two categories of demands from among many others, including assisted suicide, cultural representations, and recognition of sign language, which do not fall neatly into those two categories (Barnartt and Scotch, 2000). This paper examines the content of those demands and analyzes the implications those demands should have on social work practice.

Demands made within protests [which are one type of social movement action] are motivated by demands for change and are derived from a belief system or "collective consciousness." Such belief systems consist of ideas that transform perceptions and ultimately legitimate opposition to existing cultural beliefs or social structural arrangements (Mueller, 1987). A collective consciousness provides a lens through which a person's existence can be newly viewed and thus reinterpreted (Katzenstein, 1997: 8). It identifies a problem, suggests a solution, invokes the necessity for collective action (Klein, 1997: 23), and impels its adherents to take that action. It provides a social movement with "justification, direction, weapons of attack, weapons of defense, inspiration, and hope" (Blumer, 1995: 73). Some scholars prefer the term "oppositional consciousness" because the problem identification, explanatory framework, and proposed solutions suggested by a collective consciousness will be in opposition to the cultural explanations with which those activists were raised (Groch, 1994). It is this oppositional consciousness that makes people angry enough to engage in potentially risky contentious political actions such as protests.[3]

THE CONTENT OF DISABILITY CONSCIOUSNESS ACROSS ALL IMPAIRMENT TYPES

What is it that disability activists have been protesting about since 1970? What is the content of their collective consciousness? Most basically, it has been based upon a demand that a new model of disability be accepted by society. (See Kleinfield, 1977; Meyerson, 1988; Stroman,

1982; Deegan, 1981; Barnartt, 1986; Barnartt and Christiansen, 1985; Christiansen and Barnartt, 1987; Gleidman and Roth, 1980; Hahn, 1985a, 1985b.) These emphasized that lower incomes, economic discrimination, and political powerlessness characterize people with impairments in the same way that they characterize members of other minority groups. What was demanded was what sociologists call a frame extension (Snow, 1982; Snow et al., 1986). This involves the removal of three aspects of the cultural lens through which people with impairments have traditionally been viewed–disability as sickness, disability as deviance, and disability as an individual problem–and the application of frame of civil rights (Altman and Barnartt, 1993). In the oft-quoted title of Scotch's (1984) book, advocates wanted a change "From Good Will to Civil Rights." If civil rights were to be given to blacks, women, and others, people with impairments wanted those rights to be given to them, also.[4]

What exactly does civil rights for people with impairments mean? Central to demands by people with impairments for civil rights are (1) accessibility, which would permit the full integration of people with impairments (2) equal opportunity and (3) independent living.

Accessibility

The relative importance of the first two issues is a little different than it was for groups such as blacks or women. While equal opportunity is important, it often cannot be achieved without achieving the prior demand–accessibility. That is, if one cannot even get into the building in which the job interview is being held, one cannot have an equal opportunity to be hired for the job. Thus, civil rights for people with impairments has to include accessibility as a basic demand. There are several types of accessibility.

Architectural Accessibility

The ability to get into a building and the freedom to move within that building are the essence of architectural accessibility. People with impairments demand the right to get into public, commercial, and governmental buildings; to travel freely within those buildings; and to know where they are traveling within those buildings. Being able to get into a building may involve having a ramped or flat entrance rather than steps, having a doorway wide enough to accommodate a wheelchair, having no thresholds in the doorways, having smooth floors rather than carpets, and having automatic doors or other features (such as handles instead of doorknobs) which permit someone to be able to open them and enter.[5]

Once inside a building, other accessibility issues arise. A wheelchair user must be able to go into offices, bathrooms, bathroom stalls, and all other areas in order to have a level of access equal to that of a person who does not use a wheelchair. Wheelchairs can easily be hindered by raised thresholds as well as by types of flooring materials that make it more difficult for the wheels to move. Floors that can only be reached by steps are inaccessible to someone using a wheelchair. Heights of counter tops in a reception area; faucets, sinks, and towel dispensers in a bathroom; or switches or desks in a work area is a factor that affects the accessibility of inside areas for wheelchair users. Labels or signs are an issue for people who are blind. Braille signs or auditory indicators on items such as bulletin boards, elevator floor signals, and office labels are needed to give blind people the same information available to sighted people. In an accessible building, then, people with impairments have the same ability to move around as do people without impairments. To the extent that there is a free flow of people, those people may be both with and without impairments.

Transportation Accessibility

People with impairments demanded the ability to use public transportation systems on the same basis as people without impairments. Transportation accessibility has to do not with where people sit on a bus but with whether they can get on the bus at all–and whether they know when to get off. Buses need lifts, stations need elevators, airports need ways that permit people who use wheelchairs to get to and from airplanes, and cities may need efficient paratransit systems if they cannot provide buses with lifts and stations with elevators.

But there are also communication accessibility issues within transportation systems for people who have visual or hearing impairments. Information about times and places of arrivals and departures, both within stations and within vehicles, must be presented visually as well as aurally. Announcements of upcoming stations, schedule changes, equipment changes or breakdowns, or emergencies must be presented in both modalities. Communications using TDDs [telecommunication devices for the deaf] must be possible with ticket agents, and recorded announcements must be made available for TDD callers as well as for voice callers. Many aspects of transportation accessibility were mandated by the ADA, and there has been substantial in this area. However, lack of transportation access remains an issue for some people with some types of impairments.

Communications Accessibility

People who have hearing or speech impairments demand communications accessibility. An environment that has communication accessibility has a lack of barriers to, and therefore access to, visual or auditory communication. Communications accessibility permits people who have hearing or speech impairments to be able to express themselves in the manner they choose with the assurance that they can be understood. Communications accessibility not only includes the removal of barriers that prevent access by the person with the impairment, as is the case with architectural barriers, but it also includes removal of barriers that prevent the flow of information between people with and without impairments.

Communications accessibility requires both proximal and distal accessibility. Proximal communication takes place through written or spoken words, through voice synthesizing equipment, or through the use of interpreters or captioning (either real-time or installed). Interpreters can either be sign language interpreters, who translate from spoken language to sign language or vice versa, or oral interpreters, who relay spoken language to a person sitting quite close to them. Communications accessibility for distance interactions permits communications to take place through equipment, such as phone amplifiers, TDDs, or FM-loop systems, which permit all parties to send and receive information directly in a modality that they can interpret. Accessible distal communication can also occur indirectly using a telephone relay system, in which a third party can type words onto a TDD for the deaf person or read words from a TDD for a hearing person. E-mail and other types of computer-based communications have improved communication access for deaf people–although they may pose accessibility issues for people with visual impairments.

In a workplace, complete and ideal communications accessibility would mean that all work-, safety-, and personnel-related information would be communicated through a modality that the worker with an impairment could understand. Information in all events, including training sessions, staff meetings, office parties, and water fountain gossiping sessions, would be accessible. Off-site work, such as interviews, presentations, or professional meetings, would be equally accessible for all participants. Complete accessibility of a professional meeting for a hard-of-hearing or deaf person would include the same choice to attend or not attend sessions or to change sessions in the middle that a hearing person would have, instead of limiting the person to specific times or sessions for which interpreters are scheduled. All personnel, including coworkers and supervisors, would be able to communicate with, and to understand the communications of, the worker who has an impairment.

Communications accessibility in education would involve the ability for instructors and other students to be able to communicate with, and understand, students with hearing or speech impairments. Classroom interactions would be accessible, so that no student would ever be told, "Oh, just read the book." In addition, extracurricular activities, dorms, advising offices, and all other aspects of student life would be equally accessible to students with or without impairments.

Although access is a civil right sought by people with all types of impairments, impairment groups are sometimes divided on how best to operationalize the concept in some situations. Communications accessibility is a very different issue than architectural or transportation accessibility. Sometimes a change that meets the accessibility needs of one group might interfere with the accessibility needs of another. For example, curb cuts help people who use wheelchairs but they pose some difficulty for blind people. Having auditory announcements of subway station stops helps people with visual impairments but not people with hearing impairments.

Many aspects of communication and environmental accessibility, including state telephone relay systems, television captioning, curb cuts, and Braille signage, were mandated by the ADA or other laws. But there are still parts of society which either are not touched by these laws or which have not acceded to them, and so protests which make these demands persist. We have tried to elucidate the demands here, because it is helpful to understand them at a deeper level, since satisfying the legal demands, and satisfying demands made by individuals, is something that social workers need to work towards.

EQUAL OPPORTUNITY

The demand for equal opportunity as one component of civil rights for people with impairments is similar to demands made by blacks or women in their pursuit of civil rights. Equal opportunity means that people are not held back by characteristics such as race, sex, or impairment status in their pursuit of the good life. In a phrase heard often, people with impairments demand "a level playing field."

However, Burgdorf (1984) argues that the goal for racial and ethnic groups (as well as for women) was to make the laws as neutral as possible–to force the laws to disregard race (or sex) as a relevant classification. For people with impairments, however, neutrality may not be the most appropriate legal goal: The goal may be to *remove* barriers rather than simply ignoring them. Demands for equal opportunities for people with impairments tend to focus on work and education.

Work

In the area of work· people who are already working, who are looking for work, or who want to look for work demand nondiscrimination. As is the case for blacks or women, people with impairments demand that there be no discrimination based upon impairment status in advertising, hiring, promoting, firing, or any other aspect of employment. However, people with impairments sometimes have additional needs that must be met if equal opportunities are truly to be equal. A person might need the provision of an FM loop system for use during meetings, as well as a rule that makes sure that every speaker talks into the microphone that sends information to the user's hearing aid. Another person might need the installation of a ramp into the building, and another might need to be able to take extra rest breaks but then make up the time by working longer hours.

The presence of adequate and accessible transportation and education are related to the ability to work. If a person cannot walk or drive to work or be driven, and if the public transportation system is not accessible or if a transit system is expensive or unreliable, that person cannot get to work. Thus, demands for accessible public transportation systems are also related to demands for equal opportunity in the area of work. In addition, if educational opportunities equal to those for persons without impairments are not available to persons with impairments, they will not be able to compete equally for jobs.

Education

Many advocates feel that equal opportunity for children with impairments should mean, as it does for black children, that separate is inherently unequal. The concept of integration, when applied to children from racial or ethnic minority backgrounds, means that they should be able to attend any public school and that the same rules for school and class assignments should apply to all children. For children with disabilities, the parallel notion is that they should be educated in integrated classrooms or in the least restrictive environment at public expense. In the United States this is called *mainstreaming* or *inclusion*.

As with work-related demands, however, the situation relating to the education of children with impairments is not exactly the same as the integration of children of different racial backgrounds, so the specific demands are slightly different (Barnartt and Seelman, 1988). One demand is that children with disabilities have the right to a "free" and "appropriate" education. In this case, free means that it will be paid for by the government, no matter what the cost. As children without impairments are educated at public expense, so should children with impairments be. Appropriate means that children should be educated in "the least restrictive environment." If that environment is a regular class in a public school, or a special class in a public school, that is where the child should be educated. If that environment is a private school, a segregated day school, or a segregated residential school, that is where the child should be educated.

Although the majority of the disability community supports the demand for mainstreaming, there is not complete agreement about this demand. In particular, there is a split between advocates for children with physical (primarily mobility) impairments and advocates for children with hearing impairments. The former are strong advocates for mainstreaming; the latter are not. Many leaders in the deaf community support sending deaf children to segregated programs or residential schools rather than to schools where mainstreaming is practiced. They believe that, in reality, the least restrictive environment for those deaf children for whom ASL is their native language is one in which the child can communicate with everyone using that language, one in which deaf adults can serve as appropriate role models, and one in which the culture of deafness is taught to every deaf child (Lane, 2002).

Independent Living

A set of demands which affects many, but not all, people with impairments centers around the ability to live independently. The concept of independent living for people with impairments began when the University of Illinois began to make it possible for returning World War II veterans with impairments to attend college. It attracted more attention when Ed Roberts demanded, in the early 1960s, that the University of

California at Berkeley let him attend. In 1972 Roberts founded the Berkeley Center for Independent Living. Funding for independent living centers was included in the Rehabilitation Act of 1973, and this spurred the growth of such centers around the country.

Advocates of independent living demand that society should make it possible for people with impairments to live independently. They should not be forced to live in institutions because they need care that only an institutional setting could offer them. Rather, they should be able to live in a community of their own choosing, in a residence of their own choosing, work at a job of their own choosing if they can, and associate with people of their own choosing. They note that assistance outside of institutions costs less than the same assistance given inside an institutional setting–and it might permit some people with impairments to become tax-paying citizens.

These demands revolve around choice, self-determination, and self-actualization. People who live in institutions are told what to do and when, where, and with whom to do it. They are put in child-like and dependent positions, consistent with the sick role they are assumed to be in. Some younger people with impairments live in nursing homes, because that is the only way they can get the assistance they need for daily living activities. Independent living advocates are fighting this type of life. They argue that, if society is willing to use Medicare funds to keep people with impairments in institutions, it should be willing to spend that same money keeping them out of institutions. This could be accomplished if people with impairments had personal assistant services. Personal care attendants should be available to assist them with those tasks of daily living that they cannot do for themselves, including turning over in bed, getting dressed, bathing, eating, driving, house cleaning, and shopping. These advocates argue that people with impairments who have this kind of assistance can work and be contributing, tax-paying citizens. Furthermore, they should be the bosses who are able to hire and fire their own attendants.

These activists are demanding a reconfiguration of disability policy (Ascher et al., 1988; DeJong, 1983; Zola, 1983), which, at both the federal and state levels, has traditionally focused on income support and medical and vocational rehabilitation (Berkowitz, 1979; Liachowitz, 1988; Stone, 1984). Their concern is less with extending the frame of rights than it is with "day-to-day life and making decisions that lead to self determination" (Pelka, 1997: 166). They want people with impairments not to have to live out the sick role but to be able, with assistance, to live out a "well" role. Faced with a person with an impairment who had a job but no accessible transportation, independent living activists would want to assist that person in obtaining usable transportation, while disability rights activists would take action to make local transportation accessible to that person and all others as a matter of "rights." As Pfeiffer (1988) notes, the independent living movement is concerned with providing services that will make it possible for people with impairments to function independently.

In part, this movement is challenging the professional domination of professional in the fields of medicine, rehabilitation, psychology, social work, and related fields. As such, it is related to social movements such as the patients' rights movement, the consumers' rights movement, and the self-help movement (DeJong, 1983; Pelka, 1997: 61), all of which have similar demands. Thus the implications for social work must be considered, as we will do at the end of this article.

IMPAIRMENT SPECIFIC DEMANDS

Disability protesters comprise a somewhat unusual social movement. While most social movement have fractures and schisms, the social movement[s] occurring within the disability community are somewhat unusual in that some demands are made which refer to all people, but other demands are made which refer to a specific sub-group. In this section, we discuss those demands, which we call impairment-specific demands.

Mobility Impairments

Some of the demands made by people with mobility impairments have already been discussed with relationship to accessibility. However, there are others. One related to housing and demands the same standard of accessibility that is needed in buildings other than private homes or apartments. The types of modifications which are needed for people who use wheelchairs are seldom made in newly-built houses, even though they add very little to the cost of a new house. Retrofitting older buildings is often difficult and frequently quite costly. Therefore many public buildings remain inaccessible to people who use wheelchairs exclusively.

People with mobility–and other–impairments are demanding that all aspects of the built environment external to buildings be made accessible to them. High curbs, grassy or pebbled surfaces in parks, and even picturesque cobblestones in old cities in Europe are beginning to come face to face with demands from people with mobility impairments for curb cuts and smooth surfaces.

Deafness

In recent years, a social movement has arisen within the deaf community.[6] Some of the issues for people with hearing impairments overlap those of people demanding disability rights, especially in the area of employment discrimination. However, the specifics of accessibility and equal opportunity differ. Deaf people are not concerned with getting into a building but with being able to communicate once they are inside. They are demanding the provision of interpreters in doctor's offices, courts, and hospitals; captioning of television, movies and videos; flashing light alerting systems in hotels; TDD-accessible emergency telephone systems; and other types of communications accessibility. For deaf people, communications accessibility is the core of civil rights.

Employment discrimination issues also revolve around communications accessibility. In a workplace, deaf activists might demand provision of a TDD, an interpreter, or restructuring a job so that nonessential telephoning duties are moved to another position. Discrimination exists if, for example, a deaf person cannot understand the contents of a required training course or misses important information presented at a staff meeting because no interpreter or other communication facilitation was used.

For many deaf people, the recognition and acceptance of a deaf culture distinct from hearing culture is a major issue (White, 1998). Deaf culture is seen to have its own norms or rules for behavior, values, symbols, language, and other components. Norms include, for example, tapping someone on the shoulder, stomping on the floor, or flashing the lights in a room to get someone's attention, introducing oneself by telling one's name and where one went to school before offering any other information, and assuming that gatherings in a house will take place in the kitchen (because it usually has the best lighting). Other norms include raising and shaking hands in the air instead of clapping and standing farther apart than hearing people do when communicating in order to utilize the entire upper body for sign communication (White, 1998). There are Deaf values, including the value on signing as opposed to speaking or lipreading, a strong positive regard for ASL, rejection of the clinical-medical perspective of deafness, and a high regard for deaf children, who symbolize the continuation of Deaf culture. There are symbols, including the "I Love You" symbol and an ear with a slash through it. There are slogans, such as "Deaf people can do anything except hear," first said by Dr. I. King Jordan when he became president of Gallaudet University (Christiansen and Barnartt, 1995). There is a signed language (ASL) that contains all of the linguistic components found in auditory languages (Neisser, 1983), and one demand is that ASL be recognized as the equivalent of other languages. There is a history of the Deaf community and Deaf people that is as separate from the history of hearing people as the history of blacks is separate from the history of whites. There is Deaf humor, including a corpus of jokes passed from one generation to the next. There is also Deaf art as well as Deaf poetry (which is meant to be signed, not read) and Deaf theater. There are also items of material culture that are different for deaf people than hearing people, such as TDDs, flashing light alerting systems (doorbells, baby monitors, smoke detectors, and alarm clocks), and vibrating bed alarms.

Jankowski (1997) argues that the most basic difference between the Deaf movement and the disability movement is that the former has embraced the frames of multiculturalism and diversity rather than the frame of civil rights embraced by the latter. Under this frame, Deaf people would fight not for integration but for respected segregation. She and other activists who embrace this perspective disavow the label of disability. They see themselves as being part of a linguistic minority, not part of the disability community. For activists who accept this position, being considered to be disabled is not a compliment, and it is not an option.

It is in the area of education that Deaf activists most strongly oppose the views of people with other types of impairments. Although some Deaf people do support the concept of mainstreaming, most suggest that it has problems. Deaf students in regular schools cannot just be put into a class with other students and be expected to succeed in the same way, perhaps, that a child who uses a wheelchair might. Deaf children need additional resources. They need teachers who know how to communicate in sign language or trained interpreters.[7] In addition, because deaf students cannot watch an interpreter and take notes at the same time, students in higher grades and college classes need note takers if they are to be on an equal footing with hearing students in those classes.

But even if interpreters and note takers are provided, deaf students in hearing classrooms or schools are at a disadvantage in social interactions and extracurricular activities, for which interpreters are almost never provided. Because of this, they will have more limited opportunities to participate in sports teams or other extracurricular activities, as well as more limited social interactions,than their hearing peers. Thus, some deaf people feel that a regular classroom does not constitute a "least restrictive" environment and, in fact, may constitute the *most* restrictive environment. Those who are adamant about this situation feel so strongly that they use terms such as "communication violence" or "cultural genocide" when they discuss mainstreaming (Jankowski, 1997: 154)–and they sign it in such a way as to indicate one person being oppressed by the many. Most favor separate classrooms or, better yet, separate schools, where deaf students can interact with other deaf students and have deaf, preferable native, signing teachers in environments that address their needs for communications accessibility.

Some Deaf people also favor the continuation of separate schools because they think that this is where Deaf culture is transmitted. In these schools, Deaf culture is taught by osmosis, through role models, and sometimes explicitly, along with Deaf history, whereas in public schools with small numbers of other deaf children and no deaf adults, deaf children are not systematically exposed to either Deaf history or culture. Activists in the Deaf movement cite the demands of cultural continuation and equality in school situations in their opposition to mainstreaming.

Another reason that many Deaf activists oppose mainstreamed programs for deaf children is related to language. They feel that deaf children learn best if they learn ASL as their first, natural language and then learn written and perhaps spoken English as their second language. In that situation, English would be taught as a second language, and there would be no assumption that children would have learned it as a first language (Neisser, 1983). It follows, then, that they support the hiring of more deaf teachers and school administrators. They feel that native ASL ability is a qualification that must balance other types of academic qualifications or training when candidates for positions in schools are interviewed or hired.

A somewhat more recent demand made by the Deaf movement involves an end to the use of cochlear implants in children. Advocates of this position say that "[the procedure is highly experimental, there is no evidence that children who receive cochlear implants learn English any better than they would with conventional hearing aids or with no aid at all, and the use of an implant could 'delay the family's acceptance of the child's deafness and their acquisition of sign communication' and thus have a negative impact on the child's future quality of life in the deaf community" (Christiansen, 1998: 105-6).

Although a number of issues of communications accessibility, including the demand that each state to set up a telephone relay system, were addressed in the ADA and other recent legislation, with technological developments, new issues–and therefore new demands–have emerged. These include that digital wireless phones be compatible with hearing aids and cochlear implants and the accessibility of high-speed broadband and homeland security issues (Strauss, 2004).

Finally, independent living, and the independent living movement, is not relevant for Deaf people. They don't need personal care assistants or other aspects of independent living, and they do not participate in protests related to these issues.

Blindness

Demands related to blindness fall into several areas, one of which is transportation accessibility. Blind passengers had been denied services completely or have been hassled, intimidated, and sometimes humiliated, especially on airplanes. For example, blind passengers have been told they could not keep their white canes with them at their seats, have been denied access to exit row seating–or were arrested for refusing to sit in an exit row seat. However, the ADA and other legislation have addressed these issues.

Another set of demands relates to wages and other conditions at sheltered workshops. The Fair Labor Standards Act of 1938 encouraged the growth of such workshops for the blind, but these workers were not even paid minimum wage rates (Pelka, 1990: 282). Blind workers in sheltered workshops began to demand that wages be raised to at least minimum wage, that unemployment compensation and worker's compensation be introduced, and that the possibility of collective bargaining be permitted (Matson, 1990: 755-57).

People who are blind or visually impaired are likely to align themselves with people with other types of impairments in seeking equal opportunity and accessibility, but accessibility for them is different from accessibility for other groups. While the use of visual aids makes presentations more accessible for people with hearing impairments, if those visual aids are not also described, the presentation becomes less accessible for someone with a visual impairment. Curb cuts, which are essential for people who use wheeled mobility aids, make walking harder for blind people. Auditory indicators of elevator floors or safe street crossing times or alarm devices are useless for deaf people. Their need for personal assistants is frequently less than that of some other groups.

Psychiatric Impairments

Activists have made a number of demands for changes in treatments and other aspects of psychiatric care. One set of demands is related to promoting empowered, positive, non-psychiatric identities; the goal is "relabeling" and shedding "ex-deviant" labels (Emerick, 1991). This may be the impairment group for whom the frame-stripping part of the frame extension process is the most important. Because stigma attached to the label "ex-mental patient" (Goffman, 1963; Szasz, 1961), ex-patients seek to provide themselves with new, more positive and less deviant identities. As former patients explain:

"The way society views us is all wrong.... They then disqualify us–throw us out with the trash. Mentals [sic] are shunned, ostracized, or treated with a lack of respect. We are discriminated against, just like other minorities." Or, "Ever since I joined this [activist] group, they have got me to think differently about myself. I am no longer ashamed. It's not my fault." (Herman and Musolf, 1998: 446)

Another demand made by activists with psychiatric impairments relates to patients' rights. The most radical of the groups use terms such as "compulsory psychiatry" and call themselves "the psychiatric survivor liberation movement." These rights, they say, include an end to forced medication (Pelka, 1997: 63), an end to forced (some groups would say, *all*) electroshock treatments, an end to forced psychosurgery (i.e., lobotomies), and, overall, an end to involuntary commitment to mental hospitals. Demands relating to ending forced medication have increased with the passage of laws in some states which permit the practice. Some groups demand an end to the use of all psychotropic medication, although others think that such medicines are overprescribed but sometimes still necessary. Many groups demand an end to what they see as being tortures, including solitary confinement and tying a person to a bed, which are done in the name of treatment. Activists want mental illnesses to be considered equivalent to physical illnesses for purposes of rights and health insurance, with the end result that American culture would destigmatize mental illness.

To some extent, the demands of activists in the psychiatric survivors movement do not seem to overlap with either the disability rights movement or the independent living movement. And it is true that, in some specifics, they do not. Disability rights activists are not always attuned to the specific issues that face psychiatric survivors. And this movement sees the specific demands made by the independent living movement as having little to offer to it, since the latter's concerns are with issues of physical survival and assistance, not labeling or the right to refuse treatment.

But there are similarities. Stigmas apply to all people with visible disabilities and to those with invisible disabilities when or if those become known (Goffman, 1963). In addition, activists within the psychiatric survivors' movement applaud the extension of the frame of civil rights to people with mental as well as physical impairments. Despite the lack of overlap in specific demands, there are survivor activists who see themselves as part of the disability rights movement, and disability activists who see the psychiatric survivors' movement as part of the movement toward disability rights.

Developmental Disabilities

The earliest demands relating to developmental disabilities (which used to be called mental retardation), primarily made by parents, were related to the flagrant, severe and even life-threatening abuses that occurred in the institutional settings in which their children lived. Some of the most egregious problems have been reduced, if not solved, as a result of lawsuits and other actions brought by parents in the 1950s and 1960s. But abuses and deaths of adults with mental retardation continue to this day (see, for example, Vobejda, 2000).

Ferguson (1987) notes, however, that some of the demands made by the disability community have bypassed people with severe retardation, especially those for whom independent living is not, and never will be, possible. The minority group model, which assumes that the limitations that accompany physical impairments are due to societal practices, does not deal adequately with the situation of people with severe mental retardation. People with severe cognitive impairments will not cease to be dependent and will never live independently.

THE IMPLICATIONS OF THESE DEMANDS:
SOCIAL WORK PRACTICE
WITH PEOPLE WITH IMPAIRMENTS

These demands, and the collective consciousness they represent, suggest a number of areas and issues of which social work practitioners need to be cognizant as they interact with people with impairments.

First, the reframing of disability that is demanded implies that a disability is not a medical condition, and cannot automatically be assumed to be a disaster. Many impairments, such as deafness, cannot be treated–and many deaf people don't want their deafness to be treated. People with impairments should not be treated as children, as patients, as passive, or as dependent. One should not, for example, in the absence of other indicators, ask someone *else* what the person wants or needs.

It should be assumed that the person wants to have the power of choice. Decisions should not be made *for* someone without their input. Rather, the person should be *informed* about possibilities and *consulted* about choosing among them.

One specific area of choice involves control over services. This demand tends to be made within the context of independent living demands, especially with regard to personal assistance services. Advocates want to be able to hire, train, and fire their own pca's [personal care assistants], rather than having them provided [especially within an institutional setting]. But the demand is more general than just applying to pca's. Advocates want to be able to choose their services and their service providers.

Finally, a key implication of the reframing of disability that advocates demand is that a person with an impairment is not a child, is not sick, and should not be assumed to be, or to want to be, dependent. Services, programs, and policies need to be set up that expect and support independence rather than dependence. Thus, a policy which permits people with impairments to keep their Medicare-supported health care benefits even though they earn too much to collect SSDI benefits would support a person's being able to move toward independence, while a policy which ties Medicare to the receipt of SSDI benefits would not.

Accessibility of agencies, clinics, programs and services is of course a key demand. While it is mandated by the ADA under some circumstances, that law does not cover all situations. In particular, communications accessibility is an issue for deaf clients. It can range from the office having a TDD [and having office personnel trained to know what it is and how to use it] to the provision of qualified interpreters for meetings with deaf clients to having providers who can communicate with deaf clients in ASL and at a level the person can understand. But, in general, accessibility means that clients with impairments have the same degree of ability to take advantage of services that clients without impairments have.

Issues related to equality of opportunity may not seem to be as directly relevant to many social workers, unless they are counseling people in work or educational settings. But of course social work venues do include such settings. Additionally, many policies, including welfare, unemployment compensation, worker's compensation, and educational laws and policies are relevant to equality of opportunities for people with impairments. Overall, disability policies need to be changed to fit the new frame.

A caveat must be noted here. Barnartt and Scotch (2000) show that many protests–contrary to rhetoric–have been about services–kind, amount, location, quality, payment–and so fit a more traditional model of disability. That the disability community is not unified is clear, but that their demands are loud is also clear; these demands are changing, and will continue to change the ways in which both individuals and society interacts with persons who have physical or mental impairments.

ENDNOTES

1. Defining what is a disability issue is not easy. For the purposes of this discussion, it includes conditions which are covered under the ADA and issues which are of interest to people with physical or mental impairments. This discussion does not include protests whose sole purpose was to raise money or to celebrate disability awareness, even though those can be seen to be social movement activities.

2. See Barnartt and Scotch (2000) for extensive discussion of how information about these protests was located–although the current author has added many protests to the database discussed in that book.

3. In one-on-one situations, social workers may have to understand that the anger is part of a collective consciousness that has a positive function for social movement activity, whether or not it has a positive function for the person.

4. Additionally, activists demanded recognition that, although civil rights for blacks or women could usually be achieved for free, civil rights for persons with disabilities might cost something. Activists demand that society be willing to accept at least some cost.

5. Opening a door and entering a building may be two different things, as indicated in a recent example encountered by this author: A building had a very steep ramp to the door, and it had an automatic door opener which could be pushed by someone using a wheelchair. However, the door opened outwards, so a person getting close enough to push the automatic door opener would be pushed backwards [and down the steep ramp, probably onto their head] and could in no way enter the building.

6. People within that movement use the uppercase "D" in *Deaf* to indicate adherence to their demands; a lowercase "d" simply indicates audiological status. That is, people who are "deaf" have hearing losses but do not identify themselves as part of the Deaf community and do not support the demands made by that community (White, 1998).

7. Because of issues about correct interpretation of advanced concepts at the high school and college levels, it is crucial that the interpreter and the teacher work together to make sure that the interpretation follows the meaning of the concept rather than be a word-for-word translation.

REFERENCES

Altman, B., & Barnartt, S. (1993). Moral entrepreneurship and the passage of the ADA. *Journal of Disability Policy Studies, 4*(1), 21-40.
Ascher, G. C., Ascher, M. A., Hobbs, W. E., & Kelly, J. M. (1988). A preliminary investigation of the Independent Living Movement in Pennsylvania. *Journal of Rehabilitation, 54*(2), 34-39.
Barnartt, S. (1986). Disability as a socioeconomic variable: Predicting deaf workers' incomes. Paper presented at the American Sociological Association Annual Meeting, New York.
Barnartt, S. N., & Christiansen, J. B. (1985). The socioeconomic status of deaf workers: A minorities approach. *The Social Science Journal, 22*(4), 19-33.
Barnartt, S., & Scotch, R. (2000). *Disability protests: Contentious action 1970-1999.* Washington, DC: Gallaudet University Press.
Barnartt, S. N., & Seelman, K. (1988). A comparison of federal laws toward disabled and racial/ethnic groups in the USA. *Disability, Handicap and Society, 3*(1), 37-48.
Berkowitz, E. D. (1979). *Disability policies and government programs.* New York: Praeger.
Blumer, H. (1995). Social movements. In S. Lyman (Ed.), *Social movements: Critiques, concepts and case studies*, pp. 60-83. New York: New York University Press.
Christiansen, J. B. (1998). Cochlear implants. *Disability Studies Quarterly, 18*(2), 105-109.
Christiansen, J. B., & Barnartt, S. N. (1987). The silent minority: The socioeconomic status of deaf people. In P. Higgins & J. Nash (Eds.), *Understanding deafness socially*, pp. 171-196. Springfield, IL: Charles C. Thomas.
Christiansen, J. B., & Barnartt, S. N. (1995). *Deaf president now: The 1988 Revolution at Gallaudet University.* Washington, DC: Gallaudet University Press.
Deegan, M. (1981). Multiple minority groups: A case study of physically disabled women. *Journal of Sociology and Social Welfare, 8*(2), 274-295.
DeJong, G. (1983). Defining and implementing the Independent Living concept. In N. Crewe, I. K. Zola, & Associates (Eds.), *Independent living for physically disabled people*, pp. 4-27. San Francisco: Jossey-Bass
Emerick, R. E. (1991). The politics of psychiatric self-help: Political factions, interactional support, and group longevity in a social movement. *Social Science and Medicine, 32*(19), 1121-1128.
Gleidman, J., & Roth, W. (1980). *The unexpected minority: Handicapped children in America.* New York: Harcourt Brace Jovanovich.
Goffman, E. (1963). *Stigma.* Englewood Cliffs, N.J.: Prentice Hall.
Groch, S. (1994). Oppositional consciousness: Its manifestations and development. The case of people with disabilities. *Sociological Inquiry, 64*(4), 369-395.
Hahn, H. (1985a). Disability policy and the problem of discrimination. *American Behavioral Scientist, 28*(3), 293-318.
Hahn, H. (1985b). Towards a politics of disability: Definitions, disciplines and policies. *The Social Sciences Journal, 22*(4), 87-106.

Herman, N., & Musolf, G. R. (1998). Resistance among ex-psychiatric patients: Expressive and instrumental rituals. *Journal of Contemporary Ethnography, 26*(4), 426-449.

Jankowski, K. A. (1997). *Deaf empowerment: Emergence, struggle and rhetoric.* Washington, D.C.: Gallaudet University Press

Katzenstein, M. (1987). Comparing the feminist movements of the United States and Western Europe: An overview. In M. Katzenstein & C. M. Mueller (Eds.), *The women's movements of the United States and Western Europe,* pp. 3-22. Philadelphia: Temple University Press

Klein, E. (1987). The diffusion of consciousness in the United States and Western Europe. In M. Katzenstein & C. M. Mueller (Eds.), *The women's movements of the United States and Western Europe,* pp. 23-43. Philadelphia: Temple University Press.

Kleinfield, S. (1977). *The hidden minority: A profile of handicapped Americans.* Boston: Little, Brown.

Lane, H. (2002). Do deaf people have a disability? *Sign Language Studies, 2*(2), 356-379.

Liachowitz, C. (1988). *Disability as a social construct: Legislative roots.* Philadelphia: Temple University Press.

Meyerson, L. (1988). The social psychology of physical disability: 1948 and 1988. *Journal of Social Issues, 44*(1), 173-188.

Mueller, C. (1987). Collective consciousness, identity transformation and the rise of women in public office in the United States. In M. Katzenstein & C. M. Mueller (Eds.), *The women's movements of the United States and Western Europe,* pp. 89-110. Philadelphia: Temple University Press.

Neisser, A. (1983). *The other side of silence.* Washington, D.C.: Gallaudet University Press.

Pelka, F. (1997). *The ABC-CLIO companion to the Disability Rights Movement.* Santa Barbara, CA: ABC-CLIO.

Pfeiffer, D. (1988). Divisions in the disability community. *Disability Studies Quarterly, 8*(2), 1-3.

Scotch, R. (1984). *From good will to civil rights: Transforming federal disability policy.* Philadelphia: Temple University Press.

Snow. D. (1992). Master frames and cycles of protest. In A. D. Morris & C. M. Mueller (Eds.), *Frontiers in social movement theory,* pp. 133-155. New Haven: Yale University Press.

Snow, D. A., Rochford, E. B. Jr., Worder, S. K., & Benford, R. D. (1986). Frame alignment processes, micromobilization and movement participation. *American Sociological Review, 51*(August), 464-481.

Stone, D. (1984). *The disabled state.* Philadelphia: Temple University Press.

Strauss, K. P. (2004). Getting connected: Pressing telecommunications access issues. *SIGNews, 2*(4), 3+.

Stroman, D. F. (1982). *The awakening minorities.* Washington, D.C.: University Press of America.

Szasz, T. (1961). *The myth of mental illness.* New York: Hoeber-Harper.

Vobejda, B. (2000). City wards face daily indignities; Documents illustrate the suffering of mentally retarded in D.C. System. *Washington Post* (February 15): A1+.

White, B. (1998). From 'deaf' to 'Deaf': Defining deaf culture. *Disability Studies Quarterly, 18*(2), 82-86.

Zola, I. K. (1983). Developing new self-images and interdependence. In N. Crewe, I. K. Zola, & Associates (Eds.), *Independent living for physically disabled people,* pp. 49-59. San Francisco: Jossey-Bass.

doi:10.1300/J198v06n01_11

Applications of a Capability Approach to Disability and the International Classification of Functioning, Disability and Health (ICF) in Social Work Practice

Patricia Welch Saleeby

SUMMARY. As disability rates increase more social workers will require greater preparation to practice effectively with individuals with disabilities. The Capability approach and the International Classification of Functioning, Disability and Health provide helpful tools for social worker training. The capability approach emphasizes the need to assess what individuals are able to do in their real-life environments (capabilities) rather than capacity or functional status. The ICF provides helpful disability-related terminology and an actual classification to assist social workers to develop appropriate interventions that facilitate capability development among individuals with disabilities. Using the capability framework with the ICF will contribute to improved understanding of disability among social work students and practitioners. doi:10.1300/J198v06n01_12 *[Article copies available for a fee from The Haworth Document Delivery Service: 1-800-HAWORTH. E-mail address: <docdelivery@*

Patricia Welch Saleeby, PhD, MSSA, is Assistant Professor, School of Social Welfare, University of Missouri-St. Louis, One University Boulevard, Lucas Hall 583, St. Louis, MO 63121 (E-mail: saleebyp@umsl.edu).

[Haworth co-indexing entry note]: "Applications of a Capability Approach to Disability and the International Classification of Functioning, Disability and Health (ICF) in Social Work Practice." Saleeby, Patricia Welch. Co-published simultaneously in *Journal of Social Work in Disability & Rehabilitation* (The Haworth Press, Inc.) Vol. 6, No. 1/2, 2007, pp. 217-232; and: *Disability and Social Work Education: Practice and Policy Issues* (ed: Francis K. O. Yuen, Carol B. Cohen, and Kristine Tower) The Haworth Press, Inc., 2007, pp. 217-232. Single or multiple copies of this article are available for a fee from The Haworth Document Delivery Service [1-800-HAWORTH, 9:00 a.m. - 5:00 p.m. (EST). E-mail address: docdelivery@haworthpress.com].

Available online at http://jswdr.haworthpress.com
doi:10.1300/J198v06n01_12

KEYWORDS. Disability, capability approach, capabilities, functioning, ICF, social work practice

INTRODUCTION

According to the U.S. Census Bureau (2003), approximately 1 in 5 Americans or nearly 49.7 million people reported some type of disability or long lasting condition. The prevalence of disability is expected to increase in the United States and throughout the world due to numerous factors including accidents, aging, chronic disorders, disease, environment, land mines, malnutrition, physical abuse, sexually transmitted diseases, violence, and war (Abberley, 1987; Seelman & Sweeney, 1995). Certainly, aging of our population and the greater likelihood of developing a disability with age continue to contribute significantly to such growth.

Not only have we experienced an increase in the overall number of individuals with disabilities, there has been an increase in the percentage of individuals with disabilities living and actively participating in the community. This has resulted from three primary successful movements–namely de-institutionalization, mainstreaming, and community integration efforts. Additionally, advocacy, positive legislation, and policy advancements on behalf of individuals with disabilities have contributed. Landmark examples of such disability legislation include the Americans With Disabilities Act (1990), the Individuals with Disabilities Education Act (1975), and Section 504 of the Rehabilitation Act (1973).

Increasingly, more social workers are encountering individuals with disabilities in their respective social work clinical settings. With the growing number of individuals with disabilities living and participating in the community, a greater need for social work services provided by alternative, non-institutionalized organizations has been created. Therefore the likelihood of interaction between social workers and individuals with disabilities has increased dramatically. These trends emphasize a significant need for promoting greater awareness and training among social workers to better enable them to address disability-related issues.

Realistically, many social workers have little or no experience working with individuals with disabilities, and they have minimal exposure at the undergraduate and graduate level in most social work schools.

Social workers find themselves at a significant disadvantage to deal with these client-consumers and their disability-specific issues. Therefore, adequate exposure and preparation of all social work professionals in working with the disability population is critical for facilitating delivery of effective and appropriate services to those that require them.

AN OVERVIEW OF DISABILITY DEFINITIONS AND MODELS

Numerous definitions of disability exist in the literature but disability is generally considered difficulty in performing certain functional tasks such as seeing or hearing or activities of daily living (ADL) such as eating or dressing, or by meeting other criteria such as having a developmental or learning disability. Disability definitions have been historically negative and norm-preferred disregarding the perspective of individuals with disabilities. These traditional definitions have emphasized body and/or mind impairments and the functional limitations resulting from these conditions.

However, disability has become increasingly recognized as the dynamic interaction of the individual and his/her environment (see Table 1). While impairment is considered is a purely biological condition, disability is defined as the intersection between the demands of an impairment, society's interpretation of the impairment, and the broader societal context of disability (Braddock & Parish, 2001). As supported by the recent report, "Classifying and Reporting Functional Status" issued by the National Committee on Vital and Health Statistics, Subcommittee on Populations (2003), "functional status is affected by physical, developmental, behavioral, emotional, social, and environmental conditions. This conception encompasses the whole person, as engaged in his or her physical and social environment" (p. 2).

Similar to recent models of disability, the capability approach holds significant potential in viewing and understanding disability and functioning (Welch Saleeby, 2004; 2003a; 2003b; Welch, 2002). Developed by Nobel Laureate in Economics Amartya Sen (1987a, 1987b, 1992, 1993, 1999) with significant contribution by Martha Nussbaum (1993, 1995, 2000) the capability approach focuses on the life an individual can lead–what he/she can or cannot do and can or cannot be. Well-being is not only what an individual achieves, but also the options from which he/she has had the opportunity to choose. Capabilities represent the real opportunities an individual possesses as a result of his/her personal

TABLE 1. Examples of Common Definitions of Disability

Source	Definition
Nagi (1979)	The inability or limitation in performing socially defined roles and tasks expected of an individual within a social environment.
World Health Organization (1980) ICIDH-International Classification of Impairments, Disabilities and Handicaps	Any restriction or lack (resulting from an impairment) of ability to perform an activity in the manner or within the range considered normal for a human being.
Pope & Tarlov Institute of Medicine, IOM (1991)	The inability or limitation in performing socially defined activities and roles expected of individuals within a social-cultural and physical environment.
National Center for Health Statistics National Health Interview Survey (1992)	The state of being limited in type or amount of activities a person is expected to perform because of a chronic mental or physical health condition.
Brandt & Pope Institute of Medicine, IOM (1997)	A limitation in performing certain roles and tasks that society expects of an individual the interaction of a person's limitations with social and physical environmental factors.
World Health Organization (2001) ICF-International Classification of Functioning, Disability and Health	An umbrella term for impairments, activity limitations or participation restrictions.

ability or capacity in conjunction with his/her environment and life situation.

According to Verbrugge and Jette (1994), disability is considered "a gap between personal capabilities and environmental demand" (p. 1). Therefore, the capability approach emphasizes the need to move beyond the individual body level to understanding the influence of the environment on individual functioning and disability and the dynamic process of the individual in his/her environment. Such emphasis parallels the foundation of social work practice–specifically, the person-in-environment approach to understanding social problems and determining appropriate interventions.

AN OVERVIEW OF THE CAPABILITY APPROACH

There are two primary components in the capability approach–namely capabilities and functionings. Functionings are an individual's set of achieved doings and beings, or what he/she manages to do or to be. Capabilities are an individual's potential to achieve certain functionings, or the various combinations of what he/she can do or be. In fact, Sen equates capabilities with freedoms in that capabilities reflect the freedoms of individuals to do what they wish to do and be what they want to be (Sen, 1999). According to Sen (1987a, p. 36) "Functionings are, in a sense, more directly related to living conditions, since they are different aspects of living conditions. Capabilities, in contrast, are notions of freedom, in the positive sense: what real opportunities, you have regarding the life you may lead."

The capability approach differs from traditional mechanisms of evaluating well-being including measures of income, commodities, material goods and assets. In contrast, the capability approach recognizes that income and commodities are merely means to an end. Rather the capability approach emphasizes the importance of determining what an individual succeeds in doing with the commodities or goods at his/her command rather than the actual commodities or goods themselves. The primary reason is that individuals inherently differ from one another. Consequently, individuals differ in their ability to convert commodities and goods into capabilities and functionings.

Take two individuals who own bicycles. Individual A does not use the bicycle since he/she prefers to drive for mobility and transportation but he/she knows how and can actually ride the bicycle. This differs from individual B who does not use the bicycle because he/she was never instructed on its use, or whose parents restrict his/her usage, or who cannot manipulate the pedals due to a mobility limitation or impairment.

Recognizing the importance of interpersonal variations in the conversion process from commodities to capabilities and functionings, the capability approach places human diversity centrally in its framework and provides a more accurate depiction of overall well-being. Furthermore, in describing the factors that affect the conversion from commodities into capabilities and functionings, the capability approach facilitates a greater understanding of individual circumstances and the ability to identify potential interventions to promote capability development.

Consider the following illustration using the Welch Saleeby schematic representation of the capability approach in Figure 1. Commodities are first converted into their commodity characteristics (e.g., a manual wheelchair into its mobility or transportation properties). Although these commodity characteristics remain unaffected, the actual possession of these commodities is affected by both personal factors (e.g., adequate and available financial resources to purchase the wheelchair) and environmental factors (e.g., availability of the wheelchair commodity itself and geographical access to a wheelchair manufacturer).

FIGURE 1. Welch Saleeby Diagram of the Capability Approach

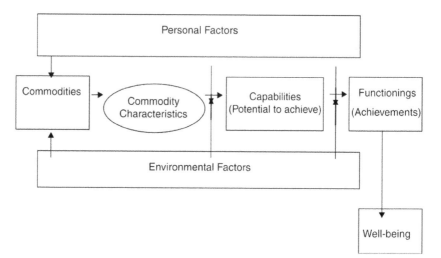

The next step is transforming commodity characteristics into capability (e.g., from the mobility and transportation properties of the wheelchair into the ability to move around, or the ability to transport oneself). This process is affected again by personal factors (e.g., severity of an individual's impairment affecting his/her ability to maneuver the wheelchair) as well as environmental factors (e.g., type of terrain or street conditions to facilitate or prevent wheelchair movement such as flat, paved roads or dirt roads with bumps). At this stage, the inclusion of the individual's environment is particularly important since it provides a more realistic assessment of what an individual can really do or his/her real potential to achieve certain functionings within the context of his/her real-life settings factoring in environmental barriers and/or facilitators.

Traditionally, only capacity or functional capacity is assessed when determining the functional status of individuals with impairments or health conditions, and it is generally measured in a standardized environment. Of course, personal factors directly affect capacity (e.g., the height or weight of an individual will affect his/her use or manipulation of certain wheelchairs and thus, adjustments are made to facilitate improved use such as raising the seat cushion). Capacity in its traditional context is only one component of the construct of capabilities. The other component is the environment since inclusion of environmental factors permits a mechanism to capture the true picture of the lived situation of individuals.

As far as what an individual actually does do or his/her functionings, these achievements are selected from the range of possible functionings, or capabilities, of that individual. The selection process is influenced by both personal and environmental factors. For example, an individual may be capable of moving around in a wheelchair in a clinical setting (capacity) as well in his/her particular actual setting (capability). Yet, he/she may be prevented from such functioning due to personal factors, such as choice or preference, religious faith, cultural values and beliefs. That individual may choose not to go outside using a wheelchair due to the perceived or actual likelihood (resulting from previous experiences) of being ridiculed by his/her peers. This would be an example of what Sen calls "constrained choice" where external forces have influenced the personal factor of choice. As a result, the environment (e.g., social forces like stigma or attitudes) plays an integral role in determining functionings by influencing aspects like choice, preference, and importance.

Accordingly, an observation of this individual's functioning level in his/her current environment may actually result in the inaccurate assumption that the individual is incapable of moving around in a wheelchair when actually the individual is capable but chooses not to do so. By comparing his/her functionings with his/her capabilities, discrepancies can be identified and a more realistic picture of the individual's lived situation is achieved. As a result, explanations for differences can be determined and interventions can be implemented to remove barriers and to promote functioning. For example, helping to improve positive attitudes and acceptance toward disabled individuals in the community is highly likely to influence an individual's choice to enter and participate in that community. By emphasizing the necessity to examine capabilities in conjunction with functionings, a greater wealth of information and understanding is gained.

Essentially, the capability approach emphasizes the need to move beyond actual functionings (outcomes or achievements) to promoting capabilities (opportunities or potential) among individuals. This is important for individuals with disabilities since traditional disability research originates from the medical model and concentrates primarily on the functioning of the individual via various functional assessments and outcome measures. Over the past decade, disability research has shifted away from focusing merely on the individual at the body level (impairment) exclusively in a clinical setting. Instead, it has moved towards understanding the contextual situation of the individual in his/her environment. Similarly, the capability approach allows us to examine both personal and environmental factors that affect converting commodities into functionings and that influence developing one's capability set.

AN OVERVIEW OF THE ICF

The International Classification of Functioning, Disability and Health (WHO, 2001) is considered by many entities as the international standard framework in describing health and health-related states. It provides a standard and unified framework to describe not only health conditions, but also to identify ways of intervening to improve the life situations of individuals with disabilities. The ICF has become increasingly supported in countries throughout the world as it has been translated into numerous languages, including Spanish, French, Dutch, Japanese, and Arabic. Moreover, it has multiple uses across sectors, including "insurance, social security, labour, education, economics, social policy and general legislation development, and environmental modification" (WHO, 2001, p. 5).

In fact, the ICF is becoming widely recognized by not only individuals and organizations in medical, health fields, and disability-related fields but other professional disciplines as well. The ICF classification has been accepted officially by the United Nations, and it is being used as an official disability definition at the international level. The ICF terminology has been incorporated in The Standard Rules on the Equalization of Opportunities for Persons with Disabilities at the United Nations. The ICF conceptual framework has been recommended as the basis for measuring disability in the United Nations Statistics Division's publication, entitled "Guidelines and Principles for the Development of Disability Statistics" (United Nations, 2002).

There has also been increased recognition of the ICF among disability representatives and organization. One example is Disabled Peoples' International (DPI), which is a network of national organizations of disabled people that promotes human rights of individuals with disabilities through full participation, equalization of opportunity, and development efforts. In its position paper, DPI proposed using the ICF as its preferred definition until its World Council develops an alternative definition. In this paper DPI states "The International Classification of Functioning (ICF) defines disability as the outcome of the interaction between a person with an impairment and the environmental and attitudinal barriers he/she may face" (DPI, 2003, p. 1). Additionally, the World Bank's Office of Disability and Development refers to the ICF as the current international guide in defining disability.

What comprises the ICF? The ICF is classified into three main components, including Body Functions and Structures, Activities and Participation, and Environmental Factors. Domains for the first component include physiological functions and structures. The second component of activities (execution of a task or action by an individual) and participation (involvement in a life situation) includes the full range of actions and life areas. However, activities relate more to the individual and participation relates more to society.

As the third component, environmental factors are the external influences on the individual with a health condition or the physical, social, and attitudinal factors that interact with the other ICF domains. Environmental factors differ from personal factors, which are also considered contextual aspects but more related to the individual's background such as age, gender, race, ethnicity, religion, social status, habits, and lifestyle. Personal factors affect an individual activities and participation, and so their contribution is recognized in the ICF framework. However, personal factors have been excluded purposefully from the classification due to their social and cultural variability.

The advantage of the ICF lies in both its conceptual framework as well as its classification. It provides an overall mechanism for preparing social workers about disability-related terminology and concepts. Additionally, it provides a classification scheme to enable social work practitioners to assess functional status, identify strengths and weaknesses, and determine appropriate interventions with their clients. Not only is the ICF a reliable and valid instrument to describe disability and functioning, it is designed for multiple uses across disciplines including social work. This is important since social workers in not only disability and health settings (hospitals, nursing homes, group homes, etc.) but in other settings (school, human services, social services, etc.) are working more with individuals with disabilities.

PARALLELS BETWEEN THE CAPABILITY APPROACH AND THE ICF FRAMEWORK

The ICF shares several common aspects with the capability approach that facilitate the use of both frameworks together. First and foremost, the ICF and the capability approach use a "biopsychosocial" approach to functioning and disability in an effort to synthesize the biological, individual, and societal perspectives of health. Consequently, both recognize the role and importance of contextual factors on individuals and differentiate between personal and environmental factors. In the ICF, environmental factors are referred to as the external influences on functioning and disability whereas personal factors are considered the internal influences on functioning and disability. The same differentiation is applied in the capability approach although slight term variations exist such as personal characteristics.

Both frameworks recognize the importance of personal factors or personal characteristics in affecting individual functioning and disability as well as their extreme variability among individuals. In fact, this is the reason the ICF purposefully does not include personal factors in its classification. In the capability approach choice as a personal factor or characteristic is considered a primary influence on determining individual functionings. Although not specifically mentioned in the ICF, choice is inherently included in the determination of what an individual actually does along with his/her ability and environment circumstances.

In the ICF functioning is the umbrella term encompassing body functions and structures, activities (the execution of a task or action by an individual) and participation (involvement in a life situation). And disability is considered an umbrella term for impairments (the loss or abnormality of bodily function and structure), activity limitations (difficulties individuals may have in executing activities), and participation restrictions (problems individuals may experience in involvement in life situations). This converse relationship of functioning and disability is similar to that of the capability approach. On one end of the continuum capability represents the ultimate combination of functionings, or the set of possible doings and beings (essentially activities and participation). On the other end of the continuum, disability represents the lack of capabilities or set of functionings influenced by factors that act as barriers.

In comparing the ICF terms to those in the capability approach (see Table 2), the ICF term participation, described as involvement in a life situation, is most comparable to the term capability, considered the ability to achieve in life. Just as capability represents the set of potential doings and beings of the individual (functioning), participation consists of the potential tasks or actions (activities) executed by an individual within his/her life context. Essentially, capability and participation both reflect the "lived experience" of individuals. Therefore, while it may be possible to assess an individual's activities and functionings in a standard environment to determine his/her capacity, it is equally if not more important

TABLE 2. Comparison of Terms and Definitions in the Capability and ICF Frameworks

	CA, Capability Approach	ICF, International Classification of Functioning, Disability and Health
Term	Disability	Disability
Definition	Deprivation of capability resulting from individual and societal factors	Restriction in participation resulting from individual and societal factors
Term	Capability	Participation
Definition	Ability to achieve in life	Involvement in life situations
Term	Functionings	Activities
Definition	An individual's doings and beings	An individual's execution of tasks

to assess an individual's performance of these activities and functionings within his/her typical or real-life environment.

Consider the activity of walking as classified under the mobility domain in the ICF. This activity is equivalent to the functioning of walking in the capability approach. It is important to determine whether an individual has the capacity or the ability to walk in the truest sense–as in a standardized testing setting such as a clinical laboratory with ideal conditions. However, it is even more important to compare this information with a determination of whether that same individual is able to walk in his/her community in real-life conditions, which may differ significantly from a standardized environment and consequently impact the individual's ability.

For example, a woman who has developed arthritis in the wrist and knee is able to walk short distances in the clinic but unable to walk in her own community due to the unleveled surfaces and unpaved roads. Consequently, she is not able to walk the five blocks to the bus stop, which is her only transportation to work. Her inability to walk eventually impacts her ability to work in an office as an administrative clerk, although her typing and filing skills are unaffected by the minor arthritis in her wrist. She is forced to quit her job and remain at home drawing benefits from the welfare system. Although a clinical assessment of capacity would not demonstrate any difficulties in walking or completing work-related tasks such as typing or filing, an assessment of performance would reveal her problems in walking in the community and most likely its effect on her opportunities for employment. Such barriers would be identified in the performance test.

As emphasized by Sen, it is imperative to look beyond an individual's functioning to his/her capability, those functionings he/she could have achieved. In doing so, one would determine the woman possesses the capability to achieve the functioning of working due to her unaffected typing and filing skills. Moreover, it is crucial to determine the reason for the gap between her achieved functioning and capability. In this case, her ability to get to work is the key element. In developing interventions to increase her participation and promote her capability, one would start by addressing her problems with transportation to work.

The comparability of terms and definitions as well as shared features between the two frameworks will certainly facilitate use of the ICF and the capability approach with each other. Bridging the capability approach and the ICF framework is a crucial step in promoting the use of both frameworks among professionals from various disciplines interested in functioning and disability. Moreover, using the ICF classification to operationalize the capability approach in addressing disability is another important component to promoting both frameworks.

USING THE ICF TO OPERATIONALIZE
THE CAPABILITY APPROACH IN SOCIAL WORK PRACTICE

The ICF provides a standard and unified framework to describe ways of alleviating and/or removing disability in conjunction with capability development efforts. As such, the ICF provides a mechanism to identify and to develop interventions that facilitate the development of capabilities among individuals with impairments or health conditions that experience disability. Different interventions are needed based upon the specific locus of disability either at the impairment, activity limitation or participation restriction levels.

Traditionally, disability has been located at the body or impairment level where the appropriate interventions are medical or rehabilitative in nature. Prevention and health promotion would be appropriate interventions for reducing or alleviating disability. Although individuals with impairments experience some loss of function or structure, they may be able to complete daily living activities without any difficulty and may not experience disability resulting directly from the impairment. However, these individuals might experience disability caused by other factors outside the individual body level in their community or society.

In these cases, societal structures, social relations, and social institutions create constraints that prevent individuals from completing daily activities, also known as the social construct of disability. Removing the disability involves intervening at an organizational and/or systems level rather than at an individual level in order to address group-dependent constraints causing the disability. Appropriate intervening tasks include removing social norms and discriminatory practices that hinder individuals with disabilities, promoting policies and legislation that address the rights of individuals with disabilities, and increasing social supports for individuals with disabilities.

At the next ICF level known as activity limitation, removing the disability involves several possible interventions to assist the individuals in overcoming their difficulties in executing activities. One mechanism uses assistive technology to compensate for activity limitations. Although assistive technology ranges from high-tech (electric powered wheelchairs, computer-assisted software, etc.) to low-tech devices (manual wheelchairs, adapted eating utensils, etc.), the crucial element is making assistive technology available, affordable, and accessible to individuals with activity limitations. Another method to address activity limitations involves rehabilitation, which attempts to correct or extend the range of individual capacities. Similarly, the important aspect involves making rehabilitation available, affordable, and accessible to individuals who need such devices. In developing countries, community-based rehabilitation has become an effective means in providing such services.

The final ICF level, participation restriction, includes interventions that change life situations. This involves removing barriers and establishing facilitators in the environment, including physical and nonphysical factors. Interventions include addressing those social and political elements necessary to facilitate environmental modification such as research, advocacy, and policy development. The availability of funding, training, and support groups are important to families of individuals with disabilities who generally serve as caregivers for those who require assistance. Additionally, education and knowledge dissemination are needed to raise awareness and change attitudes positively in communities.

Overall, the ICF offers a conceptual framework for understanding both the causes and consequences of disability. Additionally, it provides clinical information for developing appropriate mechanisms to reduce or alleviate disability and promote capabilities. As indicated in the ICF introduction (WHO, 2001, p. 6), it provides information related to "prevention, health promotion, and the improvement of participation by removing or mitigating societal hindrances and encouraging the provision of social supports and facilitators. Accordingly, using the ICF classification scheme will facilitate greater implementation of the capability framework.

CONCLUSION

There are parallels between the capability approach, the ICF, and the profession of social work that increase the likelihood of social workers using these frameworks and the associated ICF classification. One commonly used social work approach includes the "strengths perspective" which identifies individual strengths in developing mechanisms to address social problems. The ICF facilitates the ability of social workers to identify these strengths by using the ICF qualifiers, capacity and performance, along with environmental factors that act as either facilitators or barriers to individuals.

In fact, social workers generally address the individual in his/her particular environment adhering to a person-in-environment approach to social functioning and problems. As supported in the Preamble of the National Association of Social Workers Code of Ethics, "A historic and defining feature of social work is the profession's focus on individual well-being in a social context and the well-being of society. Fundamental to social work is attention to the environmental forces that create, contribute to, and address problems in living."

Overall, the capability approach and the International Classification of Functioning, Disability and Health are helpful frameworks for social work professionals to enhance their perspectives and understanding on disability. Specifically, the capability approach emphasizes the need to move beyond functionings (what individuals are doing which is influenced by choice or constrained choice) to assessing individual capabilities, essentially what individuals are really able to do or be considering their individual abilities or capacities in relation to their specific life environments. Emphasizing the need to examine both individual capabilities and functionings results in an improved understanding of the life situation of individuals and a more accurate depiction of their overall well-being.

Likewise, the International Classification of Functioning, Disability and Health offers a conceptual framework that is compatible with the capability approach, including similar terminology and key components. Additionally, the ICF classification is useful for operationalizing the capability approach, specifically in developing appropriate mechanisms to reduce or alleviate disability and improve or enhance the capabilities of individuals. Using the ICF classification scheme together with the capability theoretical framework will contribute to the improved understanding of the life situations of individuals who experience disability as well as the improved ability of social workers to deal with such issues in their clinical practices.

REFERENCES

Abberley, P. (1987). The concept of oppression and the development of a social theory of disability. *Disability, Handicap and Society, 2*(1), 5-20.
Braddock, D.L., & Parish, S.L. (2001). An institutional history of disability. In G.L. Albrecht, K.D. Seelman, & M. Bury (Eds.), *Handbook of disability studies* (pp. 11-68). Thousand Oaks, CA: Sage Publications.
National Committee on Vital and Health Statistics (2003). *Classifying and reporting functional status.* Washington, DC: Department of Health and Human Services.
Nussbaum, M.C. (2000). *Women and human development: The capabilities approach.* Cambridge: Cambridge University Press.
Nussbaum, M.C. & Glover, J. (Eds.). (1995). *Women, culture and development: A study of human capabilities.* Oxford: Clarendon Press.
Nussbaum, M.C. & Sen, A.K. (Eds.). (1993). *The quality of life.* Oxford: Clarendon Press.
Seelman, K.D., & Sweeney, S. (1995). The changing universe of disability. *American Rehabilitation, 21,* 2-13.
Sen, A.K. (1987a). The standard of living: Lecture I, concepts and critiques and Lecture II, lives and capabilities. In G.Hawthorn (Ed.), *The standard of living* (pp. 1-38).* Cambridge: Cambridge University Press.
Sen, A.K. (1987b). *Commodities and capabilities.* Oxford: Oxford University Press.
Sen, A.K. (1992). *Inequality re-examined.* Oxford: Clarendon Press.
Sen, A.K. (1993). Capabilities and well-being. In M. C. Nussbaum & A. K. Sen (Eds.), *The quality of life* (pp. 30-53). Oxford: Clarendon Press.
Sen, A.K. (1999). *Development as freedom.* New York: Alfred A. Knopf, Inc.
U.S. Census Bureau (2003). *Disability statistics 2000.* Retrieved December 5, 2004 from: http://www.census.gov/prod/2003pubs/c2kbr-17.pdf
Verburgge, L.M., & Jette, A.M. (1994). The disablement process. *Social Science and Medicine, 38*(1), 1-15.
Welch, P. (2002). *Applying the capabilities approach in examining disability, poverty and gender.* Conference proceedings, Promoting women's capabilities: Examining Nussbaum's capabilities approach, Cambridge, UK.
Welch Saleeby, P. (2003a). ICF and the social work profession. *WHO Family of International Classifications Newsletter, 1*(2), 7.

Welch-Saleeby, P. (2003b). *Disability, poverty, and development: An application of the capabilities approach in Nepal.* Conference proceedings, From sustainable development to sustainable freedom, Pavia, Italy.

Welch Saleeby, P. (2004). ICF and the capability approach. *WHO Family of International Classifications Newsletter, 2*(1), 9-10.

World Health Organization (2001). *International classification of functioning, disability and health.* Geneva: Author.

doi:10.1300/J198v06n01_12

Research Methods with Disabled Populations

Elizabeth Eckhardt
Jeane Anastas

SUMMARY. Although social work and related fields need more research involving people with disabilities, such studies can pose special challenges due to lack of understanding of disability issues, the disempowerment and invisibility of many who are disabled, and communication barriers. This article discusses ways of eliminating bias and maintaining ethical safeguards when designing and conducting research on people with disabilities. Participatory action research, which engages those studied in the design and conduct of research, is discussed as a model, as is the use of qualitative methods. Recent methodological innovations in survey research with deaf populations are also described and illustrated. doi:10.1300/J198v06n01_13 *[Article copies available for a fee from The Haworth Document Delivery Service: 1-800-HAWORTH. E-mail address: <docdelivery@ haworthpress.com> Website: <http://www.HaworthPress.com> © 2007 by The Haworth Press, Inc. All rights reserved.]*

KEYWORDS. Research methods, participatory action research, research ethics, Internet research

Elizabeth Eckhardt, PhD, LCSW, is affiliated with National Development and Research Institutes, 71 West 23rd Street, 8th Floor, New York, NY 10010 (E-mail: eae214@nyu.edu). Jeane Anastas, PhD, MSW, is Professor and Director, PhD Social Work Program, New York University, One Washington Square North, New York, NY 10003 (E-mail: jeane.anastas@nyu.edu).

[Haworth co-indexing entry note]: "Research Methods with Disabled Populations." Eckhardt, Elizabeth, and Jeane Anastas. Co-published simultaneously in *Journal of Social Work in Disability & Rehabilitation* (The Haworth Press, Inc.) Vol. 6, No. 1/2, 2007, pp. 233-249; and: *Disability and Social Work Education: Practice and Policy Issues* (ed: Francis K. O. Yuen, Carol B. Cohen, and Kristine Tower) The Haworth Press, Inc., 2007, pp. 233-249. Single or multiple copies of this article are available for a fee from The Haworth Document Delivery Service [1-800-HAWORTH, 9:00 a.m. - 5:00 p.m. (EST). E-mail address: docdelivery@ haworthpress.com].

Available online at http://jswdr.haworthpress.com
© 2007 by The Haworth Press, Inc. All rights reserved.
doi:10.1300/J198v06n01_13

INTRODUCTION

People with disabling conditions are a stigmatized group, and they are often dependent to some degree on others, people or institutions, for support and care or for other resources to support their independent living. In addition, the ways in which they function may affect the communication processes inherent in research activities. This article will address approaches to research with disabled populations, especially survey research, that can help to eliminate bias from studies and that can enhance the participation of disabled people themselves in research. It will also address data collection and ethical issues particular to the conduct of research with disabled populations, most often using illustrations that come from research within the deaf community.

An article on disabilities research could of course address the many gaps in our empirical knowledge about people with disabilities, their ways of coping and thriving, and effective methods for providing services to those who need them. It might also consider the research methods that have been and might be used with this population. However, such a review of the state of our empirical knowledge about these topics is beyond the scope of any one book chapter. This article instead has a more modest goal: to be a resource for those who might be embarking on research about and with people with disabilities. Finally, the emphasis will be on people with disabilities other than psychiatric ones, the inclusion of which would require addressing the whole field of mental health research about people with serious and persistent mental illness, some of whom are disabled by their illness.

DETECTING AND ELIMINATING BIAS

While the detection and reduction of bias is a concern in all research, it is handled in different ways in different research traditions. Traditional positivist views of research suggest that investigator bias can be eliminated, primarily through adherence to standardized and invariant methods in the conduct of the research as well as through the constant use of peer review and critique within specific scientific communities. By contrast, the view in qualitative traditions, in which the investigator's disciplined subjectivity is a tool of the research, is that bias regulation is achieved through bias recognition, although this is not to say that there is no attention to rigor and reliability in these methods (see for example Drisko, 1997, Padgett, 1998). Current views of science, which for helping professions means the research activities within them, emphasize that research, like any human activity, is historically, culturally, politically and socially situated. Therefore, standardized research tools and procedures, peer review processes, and investigator efforts at bias recognition, although all necessary, can only result in a time-specific approximation of "truth."

Bias, which is defined as systematic "error" in research results, can also arise from the theories or conceptual frameworks that guide the research. For example, early research on adult development was done on men but its findings were generalized to women as well. Similarly, current theorizing about human development assumes being able-bodied; it also assumes that average rather than facilitating or prophylactic environments are enough to sustain an individual's development and functioning throughout the life course. A deficit model of thinking about disability, for example, will point towards some aspects of functioning and some areas of inquiry as opposed while a focus on enabling environments will point to others. For example, in the case of deafness, there are obvious differences between viewing deafness as defining only a lack of ability to hear and/or to communicate in spoken language or viewing deafness as defining a culture and the use of a form of language, signing, that may have something to offer to hearing people as well, as some are suggesting for communicating with young hearing infants.

For these reasons, it is understood that bias in research is likely to be a greater problem when a study involves people and groups who are stigmatized or less powerful than others. Anastas (2000) describes several common distortions of thinking that can produce bias in research on historically marginalized groups. The first is *invisibility*, which in this case is the same as *ableism*, that is, the assumption that all research participants are ablebodied, will be answering specific questions from that standpoint, and will be able to have access to participating in the research in the usual way. This assumption can lead to segments of the population being excluded from studies altogether. Ableism can also take the form of *overgeneralization*, in which what may be true about ablebodied people is assumed to be true of those with disabilities as well. *Insensitivity* means that the possibility of disability is excluded from consideration. For example, if study participants are not asked about whether or not they have a disability, data can be distorted, as when a person with a chronic illness answers at typical item on a depression screening instrument or scale that asks about sleeping difficulties or the sense of physical wellbeing. While in an ablebodied person, such complaints may in fact suggest depression, depending on the disability or chronic condition, they might simply reflect the health reality that the respondent is dealing with. Without considering that disability or chronic illness may be salient variables to inquire about, erroneous conclusions can be drawn.

Other common distortions have to do with how research data are interpreted. *Dichotomism* occurs when differences between groups are exaggerated and similarities or overlapping characteristics are overlooked. This is another aspect of what is sometimes meant by ableism, as when people with intellectual disabilities are assumed not to have emotions or sexual needs similar to those of others, which in a research study might mean that these aspects of a respondent's everyday concerns were not asked about. *Double standards* come into play when the similar characteristics are interpreted differently in different groups. For example, again using the example of people with intellectual disabilities, the expression of sexual needs similar to those of average intellectual ability may be seen as perverse rather than normal and expectable, especially if those involved do not have access to environments affording the kind of privacy that people ordinarily seek for sexual expression. While these problems of bias can occur in any kind of research, they seem to occur most often with respect people who are socially stigmatized or who are disadvantaged in their access to social and environmental resources, as people with disabilities often are.

PARTICIPATORY ACTION RESEARCH METHODS

A model of research that strives for the empowerment of stigmatized and oppressed populations is *participatory action research* or simply *action research* (Hart & Bond, 1995; Stringer, 1999; Winter & Munn-Giddings, 2001). Action research seeks to join research, or systematic study, to the stimulation of change in the organization or social system, such as a community, being studied. Consciousness raising and the empowerment of research participants–of the groups and communities being studied–are often the hallmarks of such research. Historically, action research has been used in industrial and organizational research, in community development, and in nursing, social work and educational research (Hart & Bond, 1995). In these practice professions, its advocates believe that the use of action research can reduce the distance often observed between practice and research since its immediate aim is the improvement of practice in the research setting itself. While these strategies are often implemented in qualitative or ethnographic research contexts (see for example Stringer, 1999), elements of the approach can be used in any methodological context. One key component of action research is the deliberate inclusion of members of the communities being studied in all phases of the research, from conceptualization and planning to sampling and data gathering activities, the analysis and interpretation of a study's findings, and in the dissemination of results within the community that supplied the study opportunity and the data. For example, while it may not be indigenous members of the disabled community who have the funding and the expertise to conduct a study, those who are doing so make every effort to involve representatives of those being studied in all phases of the research. This involvement may be through employment in core roles on a project and/or through the use of consultants to a project, paid or volunteer. Such involvement must not simply be for "window dressing" but should be designed to ensure that the views of the community, or at least some of its members, are central in the activity. Research studies are invariably enriched when indigenous researchers, or at least indigenous consultants, are used–in access to samples, effective data-gathering, valid interpretation of data, and the acceptance and use of findings once a study has been completed. A later section of this chapter specifically addresses the use of members of the group being studied in the development of survey instruments.

Ethical Issues

Three basic principles underlie all ethical standards for the conduct of research with human being: *beneficence, justice* and *respect. Beneficence* means that neither individuals nor the population being studied should be harmed by participation in the research. *Justice* means that the rights of participants are respected. *Respect* means that the dignity and self-determination of research participants is safeguarded. Adhering to these principles means, for example, that research participants must give free and informed consent to involvement in research and that there must be no coercion, even undue inducement, or loss of services as a result of refusal to take part in a study. Because of these principles, respecting the privacy of research participants, including their right not to be identified as research participants, must also be a major goal. Unfortunately, history shows that people with disabilities, such as those who lived in institutions for the mentally retarded, have not always had these rights respected. When a group is conscious of a history of abuse in the name of research, it can understandably lead a collective to mistrust of research activities even in this era of systematic oversight of research via institutional review boards, which may be true in some disabled populations.

When conducting research with people with disabilities, there are often special issues to consider when obtaining informed consent. Research participants must understand the information presented to them in a consent document, and it is the researcher's ethical responsibility to ensure that they do. In research with the Deaf, this can mean translating informed consent documents into the participants' native language, such as ASL. A study that used a computerized self-administered instrument to assess mental health provides an example of this kind of procedure (Eckhardt, Steinberg, Lipton, Montoya & Goldstein, 1999; Steinberg, Lipton, Eckhardt, Goldstein & Sullivan, 1998). In some cases, information from the informed consent was signed in ASL by a member of the research team and each participant was asked to communicate the information back in ASL, all in the presence of a witness fluent in ASL to insure that the potential participant had understood the content of the consent form. Not until all parties agreed that each participant understood the content were participants asked to provide their signature. In other instances, Institutional Review Boards required the informed consent documents be videotaped in ASL as a way to insure that participants from their institutions fully understood their content, including all the risks and benefits of participation in the study.

Many ethical dilemmas in web-based research have not yet been adequately addressed (Rhodes, Bowie, & Hergenrather, 2003). What constitutes an adequate indication of consent? What if the anonymous respondent is a minor, from whom one would otherwise have to seek parental consent for participation? Finally, in other survey research with vulnerable populations, there are often protocols in place should a research participant demonstrate distress during the conduct of the research, but such precautions may be very difficult to implement in web-based research. As ethical standards for web-based research evolve, standards of practice for addressing these potential problems will become clearer.

Sampling and Recruitment

When conducting research with individuals who are disabled, it is important to have well-defined sampling criteria. For example, when conducting research with a deaf population, it is important to determine whether you are interested in learning about individuals who are prelingually deaf, who communicate primarily using ASL; in deaf individuals who are considered oralists and use speech, reading and voice to communicate; or both. You may want to include individuals who were deafened later in life and/or those who consider themselves hard of hearing. In addition, you may be interested in doing a study on those who consider themselves culturally Deaf, in which case you may not be able to include all individuals who are deaf, hard of hearing, or hearing impaired. Such decisions, which should be based in the purposes of the research, have implications both for who you will recruit to the study and for how the data gathering will be conducted.

Because there are no population-based lists of those who are deaf or hearing impaired, random sampling is not possible since no sampling frame exists. In addition, although the long form used in the nation Census includes some questions about disabilities, including sensory difficulties, because there is no single widely accepted definition of deafness, the number of deaf individuals in any given geographic area is poorly documented (Schein, 1987). Therefore, other sampling strategies, such as purposive, snowball and targeted sampling, must be used. Lipton and Goldstein (1997) employed targeted sampling techniques when recruiting for a substance use study. Targeted sampling involves inviting individuals (in the absence of any list) who are present on the street, at an event, or in organizations to participate in a study. When seeking deaf study participants, large service organizations, deaf recreational programs, and deaf sports leagues were used by Lipton and Goldstein (1997), who were able to obtain a sample of over 800 for their study.

As the internet becomes a more common medium for research, it is important to consider the nature of samples obtained in this way (Rhodes, Bowie, & Hergenrather, 2003). Web-based survey research certainly has the potential to reach across geographical boundaries and to reach hidden populations, and the anonymity of the medium may in fact encourage honest responses to sensitive questions. However, response rates have been the traditional measure of sampling adequacy in mailed and telephone surveys, and response rates cannot be calculated for Web-based surveys. In addition, although some precautions can be taken to reduce the problem, multiple responses from the same respondent can also be a problem. Finally, the "digital divide" still exists, excluding people without computer or web access from participation in such research, and literacy levels must also be considered. However, technological advances that make the use of computers possible for those with disabilities continue, such as speech systems and pointers with touch screens, which suggests that use of the web for disability research is likely to grow.

Data Collection

The importance of participation from the targeted disability group(s) in all phases of research cannot be overstated. This section will focus on the following factors related to data collection when conducting survey research with individuals with disabilities: determining methods of data collection to maximize accessibility; determining whether to adapt existing surveys used with the general population or to develop new surveys specifically for use with individuals with disabilities or specific disability groups; and the importance of including individuals with disabilities in survey development.

Data Collection Options

Researchers must determine what will be the most effective method(s) of collecting data from the targeted disability group(s) for maximizing accessibility to all individuals. Most researchers choose standardized surveys with closed ended questions when attempting to collect data from large numbers of individuals. Standardized surveys are valuable because they insure that each respondent is answering the same question. In survey research, options include self-administered written surveys, face to face surveys administered by a trained interviewer (may include the use of proxies for responses), computer assisted surveys, self-administered computer surveys (including internet surveys), and telephone surveys.

There are several factors to consider when determining the best method(s) of data collection to use when surveying individuals with disabilities. For a survey that seeking a representative sample of individuals with disabilities, often multiple methods of data collection are used. The Bureau of Transportation Statistics, U.S. Department of Transportation developed and conducted a transportation survey targeted to people with disabilities. The survey was made available for completion via telephone interview by trained interviewers (many with disabilities themselves), in writing to be mailed to the respondent, and on-line via the computer (Durant, 2004).

In making these decisions, researchers must assess whether targeted respondents can read or hear the questions, and whether they are able to signal their response themselves. A study conducted to determine the inclusion of people with disabilities in the National Household Interview Survey assessed the use of proxy response (Kaye, 2004). This study concluded that people with very severe physical disabilities rarely responded for themselves (as inferred from the level of assistance needed for activities of daily living), with the majority of these individuals using assisted response measures. For individuals with cognitive impairments such as Alzheimer's or mental retardation, more than 60% used proxy response. This study also concluded that 50% with severe speech impairment used proxy response, while (62%) of individuals who are deaf used self report, 63% of people with mobility impairments used self-report, and 65% of individuals who are blind used self-report as did approximately 60% of individuals with mental illness.

When conducting surveys with individuals who are deaf and whose primary communication modality is ASL, there are several factors that must be considered when determining the best method for collecting data. For example, the lack of literacy skills in the profoundly and pre-lingually deaf population makes it difficult for them to be fairly tested with a *written* questionnaire (Gordon, Stump, & Glaser, 1999; Marschack, 1993). In addition, direct interviewing by non-signing professionals without an interpreter is not possible because, on average, the deaf adult will not understand more than 26%-40% of one-to-one conversation through lip-reading (Gordon, Stump, & Glaser, 1996; Waldstein & Boothroyd, 1995). Zazove et al. (1993) report that the expectation on the part of health care providers that all deaf individuals can write, or lipread has resulted in frustration for both the deaf individual and the health care provider.

Confidentiality is a real problem for individuals who are deaf, in terms of both the risk to the individual and the individual's reluctance to communicate during interviews conducted with interpreters where sensitive issues are explored (MacDougall, 1991). Although certified interpreters have a strict code of ethics that mandates confidentiality, impartiality, discretion, and maintenance of professional boundaries, individuals who are deaf often express concern about discussing subjects such as medical symptoms in the presence of such an interpreter (MacDougall, 1991; Steinberg, Sullivan, & Leow, 1998; Vernon & Miller, 2001). This problem is magnified when certified interpreters are not available and when less well-trained signers (who may not fully understand the implications of the strict code of ethics) or a friend or family members are asked or offer to help. These problems are exacerbated in communities with few trained interpreters. When the individual who is deaf anticipates future contact with the interpreter in other settings, a sense of true privacy cannot be achieved.

Some instruments, for example, the WISC-III used to test intelligence, or the SCID used in mental health testing, require the person administering the test to interact with the individual being tested. Even if this is done one-on-one with ASL, there is no standardization of the actual sign translation. American Sign Language is a complete language unto itself, it is not English. There is no *standard* written format for ASL or its English-based sign variants (Woodroffe, Gorenflo, Meador, & Zazove, 1998). Therefore each signer administering the test is likely to translate the same English sentence somewhat differently.

Technology has offered solutions to some of the difficulties in making sure that all individuals with disabilities have full access to participation in surveys. Web-based surveys have brought the research into people's homes, schools, and other organizations. There are benefits to this in that a respondent has the freedom to complete the survey at his or her own pace, and it is cost-effective because the need for field workers is reduced, cutting down on overall data collection costs. While Web-based surveys are becoming more popular, it is important to recognize that there are still many individuals who lack computers and/or Web access, limiting the generalizability of findings generated in this way.

Technology has certainly helped some researchers achieve greater access to individuals who are deaf and who use ASL as their primary mode of communication. Specifically, the use of interactive video and computer technology has enabled researchers to develop health-related surveys and screening instruments that are self-administered in ASL. Social Science Innovations Corporation has used these techniques to develop a measure of substance use in a sample of 850 deaf adults (Lipton & Goldstein, 1997; Lipton, Goldstein, Fahnbulleh, & Gertz, 1996); a mental health assessment instrument (Eckhardt et al., 1999); a tobacco use questionnaire used with youth in the Los Angeles area, conducted in collaboration with the University of California Tobacco-Related Disease Research program (Berman et al., 2000); and currently an HIV Knowledge, Attitudes and Beliefs survey for use with Deaf adults (Goldstein, Eckhardt, Joyner & Berry, 2004). These surveys have been conducted primarily using laptop computers that are brought to data collection sites.

USE OF EXISTING SURVEYS
VERSUS DEVELOPMENT OF NEW SURVEYS

Some researchers grapple with the decision of whether to adapt standardized surveys which were developed for use with the general population or to develop new surveys to be used specifically for use with individuals with disabilities. Researchers often prefer to use existing instruments because they allow for comparison of results with the general population. While it is beneficial to use existing surveys for this reason, there are several questions a research team should answer before determining whether to use an existing survey with adaptations and additions or whether to develop a new survey specifically for the topic and disability group of interest. These questions include:

1. Are survey items relevant for the disability group(s) being researched?
   For example, some health related surveys may inquire about cardiovascular exercises, including running, walking, climbing stairs, etc., and individuals in wheelchairs may find these questions offensive or may answer in a way that skews the results.
2. Are the questions asked in a language that is accessible to the targeted sample?
   Many deaf adults read between the third and fifth grade levels (Gordon, Stump, & Glaser, 1999). Even for those proficient in English, if American Sign Language is their first and natural language, surveying these individuals in written English would not yield optimal results.
3. Is there information specific to the disability group that you are researching that cannot be obtained using the existing survey?

To illustrate, most HIV/AIDS information and prevention instruments are available only in written forms. Although a small minority of people who are post-lingually deaf as well as those deafened later in life may respond to English-based questionnaires, many pre-lingually deaf individuals find these instruments confusing and misleading (Steinberg 1991). This is due partly to the reading level–most surveys and questionnaires are written in 9th grade English, while most pre-lingually deaf persons read substantially below this level (Kennedy & Bucholz, 1995; Vernon & Miller, 2001). In addition, when interviewing individuals who are deaf about their knowledge, attitudes and beliefs about HIV/AIDS, some important questions about the sources of information (deaf schools, hearing schools, work shops conducted in ASL) may not have been included in surveys used with the general population.

Researchers will often decide to use existing surveys but to adapt these surveys for their research. For example, researchers at the University of Illinois-Chicago developed an Internet survey that questioned mental health consumers about their personal experiences of self-determination, feelings about the service delivery system, and their use of information technology. This survey incorporated items from the U.S. Bureau of the Census technology survey, the Pew Internet Life Project, and added other items of interest (Cook, Fitzgibbon & Batteiger, 2004). For an HIV/AIDS Knowledge, Behaviors, and Attitudes Survey developed for use with deaf adults (Goldstein et al., 2004), questions were chosen from the National Health Interview Survey (1998) and the HIV-Knowledge Questionnaire (Carey et al., 1997), each used with the general population, and from a written HIV/AIDS questionnaire for a deaf sample (Woodroffe et al., 1998). Deaf specific questions were also added to the survey including demographic questions, such as, how do you identify yourself (deaf or hard of hearing), sources of information, and some questions about HIV testing and confidentiality issues.

These studies employed rigorous translation procedures to ensure cultural sensitivity and linguistic effectiveness. Generally accepted guidelines for translating research questions between two languages (Brauer, 1993; Edwards, 1994; Phillips, Hernandez, & Ardon, 1994) were employed. Techniques used to attain translation equivalence included back-translation, decentering, and a translation team approach (Eckhardt et al., 1999; Edwards, 1994; Phillips, Hernandez & Ardon, 1994; Montoya et al., 2004). Back translation is a process for assessing whether a translation in accurate; a bilingual individual who has not seen original text translates the new translation back into the original language. Decentering is the iterative process of translating to the target language, back-translating to the source language, and negotiating the modification of both the source and the target language as needed so the original construct is as conceptually, linguistically and operationally equivalent in both languages as possible. In these studies, a translation team approach was used consisting of a team of individuals who were Deaf and in some cases hearing, who were fluent in ASL and who had extensive knowledge working with different subgroups within the Deaf community. An expert in ASL was also used to review translations and provide feedback and suggestions on them, and the ASL expert was also called upon for consultation when there was disagreement on the translation team regarding the most effective translations. For detailed descriptions of the translation procedure and to review some of the translation challenges inherent in translating a mental health diagnostic instrument from written English into ASL, see Eckhardt et al. (1999) and Montoya et al. (2004), which highlight the special considerations and rigor such research necessitates.

USE OF MEMBERS
FROM THE TARGETED DISABILITY GROUP
IN SURVEY DEVELOPMENT

In addition to having individuals with disabilities on the research team, focus groups comprised of individuals from the targeted group are often used in the survey development phase (Eckhardt et al., 1999; Montoya et al., 2004; Cook, Fitzgibbon, & Batteiger, 2004; Durant, 2004). The use of focus groups is helpful in determining which items to include and which to omit from existing surveys, how to adapt or translate original survey items, and what additional items may be necessary. Focus groups are also used during survey development to gain feedback from the targeted disability group regarding the content of the research. Feedback from these focus groups can help determine survey domains and may provide information related to length of survey, item layout and optimal response options.

Data analysis from six focus groups conducted during the survey development phase of the HIV/AIDS Knowledge survey for use with individuals who are Deaf revealed several themes that contributed the final computerized, self-administered HIV/AIDS knowledge survey in American Sign Language. Focus groups comprised of deaf adults from various sectors of the deaf community were shown videotaped ASL versions of potential survey items. Results from the focus groups demonstrated that there is a segment of the deaf community with minimal sign language skills who did not readily comprehend the level of ASL used for the videotaped translations. To successfully meet the needs of the greatest number of deaf individuals whose main form of communication is sign language and who are not fluent in written, spoken or signed English, it was suggested that we include two versions of ASL, one which would meet the needs of deaf individuals who have higher level ASL proficiency, and another version created specifically for the segment of the deaf population which communicates using "highly contextual" ASL. Providing these two versions of ASL made the survey more accessible all members of the deaf community. It was crucial to include accessibility to include individuals with minimal language skills because these are the individuals who have been systematically excluded from surveys due to their lack of English literacy and their level of sign language skills.

Feedback from the focus groups also influenced the format of response options. Surveys often use Likert scale response options to determine degree of knowledge or agreement, and HIV/AIDS surveys conducted among the general population are no exception. When Likert scale responses were shown to focus groups, feedback demonstrated that participants with minimal language skills and participants for whom ASL is not their original language were not familiar with this type of response option. Therefore the survey incorporated only Yes/No/Don't Know and True/False/Don't Know response options for the survey.

QUALITATIVE METHODS

As described above, qualitative methods of research, including focus groups and in-depth interviews, are vital in informing survey development. In one study, Crowe (2003) utilized focus groups comprised of deaf and hard of hearing individuals from various segments of the deaf community to develop HIV prevention material that was culturally and linguistically sensitive. The rich data from these focus groups underscored the importance of conducting focus groups comprised of individuals for whom research is targeted. Focus group participants confirmed the need for HIV prevention material for deaf individuals, provided suggestions for the design of prevention materials, and evaluated sample materials, ultimately agreeing upon the final products, in this case a poster and a condom card.

However, as paradigms of action research also suggest, qualitative methods are also very useful on their own in disability studies. Qualitative methods are especially well-suited to uncovering the nature of people's subjective experiences and for understanding a phenomenon about which little is known (Anastas, 2000; Padgett, 1998; Strauss & Corbin, 1990). They can provide details of experiences that are difficult or impossible to gather through quantitative means. For example, Nosek et al. (2004) used focus group and individual interviews with women with physical disabilities to learn how they defined health and how they engaged in health-promoting activities. One finding was that even a woman with severe impairments in mobility might define herself as healthy if she was able to perform her usual social roles and activities (even if now diminished) and if she were not suffering from any acute condition (such as a urinary tract infection), a "ceiling effect" that was also evident in how some women handled exercise goals. Health was thus defined functionally and not in the traditional sense of the absence of any disease state. These realities would not have been captured by a survey method of self-ratings of health, which would likely have been misinterpreted.

CONCLUSION

Social work practice with people with disabilities should certainly include relevant research. Studies can be aimed at needs assessment, at describing the problems and successes achieved by those with chronic illness or with sensory or motor challenges, at the evaluation of services, or at what may be needed to make environments more facilitative for everyone. Doing research is a communication process, although a specialized one, and many of the points made in this article have to do with making the communication process between researchers and other research participants effective. Doing research with vulnerable populations also means that special attention to ethical issues is necessary as well. Finally, given the ongoing shifts in how disabilities are conceptualized, the stigma attached to disability, and our current lack of knowledge about the lives of people with disabilities, involvement of those we aim to study in all levels of the research process is an imperative.

REFERENCES

Anastas, J. W. (2000). *Research design for social work and the human services, 2nd ed.* New York: Columbia University Press.

Berman, B.A., Eckhardt, E.A., Kleiger, H.B., Wong, G., Lipton, D.S., Bastani, R. et al. (2000). Developing a tobacco survey for deaf youth. *American Annals of the Deaf, 145*(3), 245-255.

Brauer, B. A. (1993). Adequacy of a translation of the MMPI into American Sign Language for use with deaf individuals: Linguistic equivalency issues. *Rehabilitation Psychology, 38*(4), 247-260.

Carey, M.P., Morrison-Beedy, D., & Johnson, B.T. (1996). The HIV-knowledge questionnaire: Development and evaluation of a reliable, valid, and practical self-administered questionnaire. *AIDS and Behavior, 1*(1), 61-74.

Cook, J.A., Fitzgibbon, G., & Batteiger, D. (2004). Self-determination and technology web survey. Presented at the, Best Practices for Surveying People with Disabilities Conference. Sponsored by the Interagency Committee on Disability Research. Subcommittee on Disabilty Statistics. Washington, DC.

Crowe, T. V. (2003). Using focus groups to create culturally appropriate HIV prevention material for the Deaf community *Qualitative Social Work: Research & Practice, 2*(3), 289-308.

Dunnett, B. (2001). Developing client-focused work with people with profound learning disabilities. In R. Winter & C. Munn-Giddings (Eds.), *A handbook for action research in health and social care,* (pp. 116-130). New York: Routledge.

Durant, S.L. (2004). "A case study on full particpation in surveys." Presented at the Best Practices for Surveying People with Disabilities Conference. Sponsored by the Interagency Committee on Disability Research. Subcommittee on Disabilty

Statistics. Washington, DC http:www.bts.gov/omnibus_surveys/targeted_survey/ Then click "National Transportation Availability and Use Survey" to access the survey documentation and public use files.

Eckhardt, E., Steinberg, M.D., Lipton, D.S., Montoya, L., & Goldstein, M.F. (1999). Innovative directions in mental health assessment Part III, Use of interactive technology in assessment: A research project. *Journal of American Deafness and Rehabilitation Association, 33*(1), 19-29.

Edwards, N.C. (1994). Translating written material for community health research: Guidelines to enhance the process. *Canadian Journal of Public Health, 85*(1), 67-70.

Goldstein, M.F., Eckhardt, E., Joyner, P., & Berry, R. (2004). HIV knowledge in a Deaf sample: Preliminary results of a self-administered survey in American Sign Language. [Abstract in press] American Public Health Association Annual Meeting, Nov. 2004: Washington, DC.

Gordon, R.P, Stump, K., & Glaser, B.A. (1996). Assessment of individuals with hearing impairments: Equity in testing procedures and accommodations. *Measurement and Evaluation in Counseling and Development, 29*, 111-118.

Hart, E., & Bond, M. (1995). *Action research for health and social care.* Buckingham, England: Open University Press.

Kaye, H.S. (2004). Inclusion of people with disabilities in the NHIS & NHIS-D: Non-response, proxy response, and assisted response. Presented at the Best Practices for Surveying People with Disabilities Conference. Sponsored by the Interagency Committee on Disability Research. Subcommittee on Disabilty Statistics. Washington, DC.

Kennedy, S.G., & Buchholz, C.L. (1995). HIV and AIDS among the deaf. *Sexuality and Disability, 13*(2), 111-119.

Law, M. (1997). Changing disabling environments through participatory action research. In S.E. Smith & D.G. Williams (Eds.), *Nurtured by knowledge: Learning to do participatory action research.* New York: Apex Press.

Lipton, D.S., & Goldstein, M.F. (1997). Measuring substance abuse among the deaf. *Journal of Drug Issues, 27*(4), 733-754.

Lipton, D.L., Goldstein, M.F., Fahnbulleh, F.W. & Gertz, E.N. (1996). The Interactive Video-Questionnaire: A new technology for interviewing Deaf persons. *American Annals of the Deaf, 141*(5), 370-378.

MacDougall, J.C. (1991). Current issues in Deafness: A psychological perspective. *Canadian Psychology, 32*(4), 612-627.

Marschark, M. (1993). *Psychological development of deaf children.* New York: Oxford University Press.

Montoya, L.A., Egnatovitch, R., Eckhardt, E., Goldstein, M., Goldstein, R.A., & Steinberg, A.G. (Summer 2004). Translation challenges and strategies: The ASL translation of a computer-based psychiatric diagnostic interview. *Sign Language Studies, 4*(4), 314-344.

Nosek, M.A., Hughes, R.B., Howland, C.A., Young, M.E., Mullen, P.D., & Shelton, M.L. (2004). The meaning of health for women with physical disabilities: A qualitative analysis. *Family and Community Health, 27*(1), 6-21.

Padgett, D.K. (1998). *Qualitative methods in social work research: Challenges and rewards.* Sage: Thousand Oaks, CA.

Phillips, L.R., Hernandez, I.L., & Torres de Ardon, E. (1994). Focus on psychometrics: Strategies for achieving cultural equivalence. *Research in Nursing & Health, 17,* 149-154.

Rhodes, S.D., Bowie, D. A., & Hergenrather, K. C. (2003). Collecting behavioural data using the world wide web: Considerations for researchers. *Journal of Epidemiology & Community Health, 57*(1), 68-73.

Schein, J. D. (1987). Deaf population: Demography. *Gallaudet encyclopedia of deaf people and deafness.* New York: McGraw Hill.

Springer, E.T. (1999). *Action research, 2nd ed.* Thousand Oaks, CA: Sage Publications.

Steinberg, A., Lipton, D.S., Eckhardt, E.A., Goldstein, M.F., & Sullivan, V.J. (1998). The Diagnostic Interview Schedule for deaf patients on interactive video: A preliminary investigation. *American Journal of Psychiatry, 155*(11), 1603-1604.

Steinberg, A., Sullivan, V.J., & Leow, R. (1998). Cultural and linguistic barriers to mental health service access: The deaf consumers' perspective. *American Journal of Psychiatry, 155*(7), 982-984.

Strauss, A., & Corbin, J. (1998). *Basics of qualitative research: Techniques and procedures for developing grounded theory.* Thousand Oaks, CA: Sage Publications.

Vernon, M., & Miller, K. (2001). Interpreting in mental health settings: Issues and concerns. *American Annals of the Deaf, 146*(5), 429-434.

Waldstein, R.S., & Boothroyd, A. (1995). Speechreading supplemented by single-channel and multichannel tactile displays of voice fundamental frequency. *Journal of Speech & Hearing Research, 38,* 690-705.

Winter, R., & Munn-Giddings, C. (2001). *A handbook for action research in health and social care.* New York: Routledge.

Woodroffe, T., Gorenflo, D.W., Meador, H.E., & Zazove, P. (1998). Knowledge and attitudes about AIDS among deaf and hard of hearing persons. *AIDS Care, 10*(3), 377-386.

Zazove, P., Neiman, L.C., Gorenflo, D.W., Carmack, C., Coyne, J.C., & Antonucci, T. (1993). The health status and health care utilization of deaf and hard of hearing persons. *Archives of Family Medicine, 2*(7), 745-752.

doi:10.1300/J198v06n01_13

Index

Ableism, 235
Accessibility, 190,197
  architectural, 197-198
  communications, 199-200
  transportation, 198-199
Action research, 236-242
Activism. *See* Disability activism
ADA. *See* Americans With Disabilities
    Act (ADA) (1990)
ADAPT (American Disabled for
    Attendant Programs Today),
    39-40
Adolescents with disabilities. *See*
    Children/adolescents with
    disabilities
Adoption Assistance and Child
    Welfare Act (1980), 114
Advocacy
  ADA and, 83-86
  skills, for people with disabilities
    and, 86-89
Albertsons Incorporated vs.
    Kirkingburg, 78-79
American Disabled for Attendant
    Programs Today (ADAPT),
    39-40
American School, of object relations
    theory, 172
Americans With Disabilities Act
    (ADA) (1990), 40-41
  advocacy and, 83-86
  background to, 68
  court rulings on, 76-80
  defining disabilities under, 78-79
  definition of disability in, 70-71
  findings supporting need for, 69
  lobbying for, 94
  people with HIV infection and, 77
  prison systems and, 77-78

purposes of, 69
social security benefits and, 77-78
titles of, 40,71-75
Architectural accessibility, 197-198
Assets, developmental, 124
Attention Deficit Disorder (ADD), 32
Attention Deficit Hyperactivity
    Disorder (ADHD), 32

Bias
  detecting/eliminating, 234-236
  distortions of thinking that can
    produce, 235-236
Blindness. *See* Vision loss
Board of Trustees of the University of
    Alabama vs. Garrett, 79-80
Bragdon vs. Abbott, 76
British School, of object relations
    theory, 172

Capability approach, 219-220
  ICF and, 225-228
  overview of, 220-224
  using ICF to operationalize,
    228-230
Change agents
  characteristics of, 96-97
  in deaf community, 97-99
Charles Wessel vs. AIC Security
    Investigation, Ltd., 81
Children/adolescents with disabilities,
    112
  families and, 125-128
  legislation for, 113-123
  siblings of, 128-129
Chronic sorrow, 9

function limitations and, 159-161
low vision and, 158-159
personal experience of, 161-170
Vouchers, for disabled people, 13

Web-based surveys, 242
Work, equal opportunity for, 201

Yeskey, Ronald R., 77

Zero reject/child find principle, of
  IDEA, 26

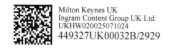